# Medical Careers
# and
# Feminist Agendas

# SOCIAL INSTITUTIONS AND SOCIAL CHANGE
*An Aldine de Gruyter Series of Texts and Monographs*
EDITED BY James D. Wright, *University of Central Florida*

# Medical Careers
# and
# Feminist Agendas

## AMERICAN, SCANDINAVIAN,
## AND RUSSIAN WOMEN PHYSICIANS

## Elianne Riska

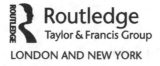

Routledge
Taylor & Francis Group

LONDON AND NEW YORK

First published 2001 by Transaction Publishers

Published 2017 by Routledge
2 Park Square, Milton Park, Abingdon, Oxon OX14 4RN
711 Third Avenue, New York, NY 10017, USA

*Routledge is an imprint of the Taylor & Francis Group, an informa business*

Library of Congress Catalog Number: 2001022600

Library of Congress Cataloging-in-Publication Data

Riska, Elianne
  Medical careers and feminist agendas : American, Scandinavian, and Russian women physicians / Elianne Riska
        p. cm. — (Social institutions and social change)
  Includes bibliography, references and index.
  ISBN 0-202-30667-4 (cloth : alk. paper) — ISBN 0-202-30668-2 (pbk. : alk. paper)
     1. Women physicians-Cross cultural studies.   2. Women physicians-United States.   3. Women physicians-Russia (Federation) 4. Women physicians-Scandinavia.   5. Women in medicine-Cross cultural studies.
  6. Sexism in medicine—Cross cultural studies. 7. Social medicine-Cross-cultural studies.   I. Title. II. Series.
R692 .R57 2001
610'.82-dc21                                                          2001022600


ISBN 13: 978-0-202-30668-1 (pbk)

# Contents

# Contents

# Preface

This monograph is the result of a research effort that was originally generated while I was teaching medical students at the College of Human Medicine at Michigan State University in the 1970s. I was intrigued by the character of the socialization process that the medical students had to undergo during their training, a process quite different from that typical in other disciplines. Ever since, I have studied and followed the changes in the status and power of the U.S. and Scandinavian medical profession. Theory and research in the sociology of professions and health sociology have shown me how knowledge is generated and organized in the modern world. In most of my work I have been interested in the sociology-of-knowledge aspect of the development of modern medicine.

My adoption of a gender perspective on the medical profession can be traced to reading Judith Lorber's pioneering book on women physicians in 1984. While I was doing the research reported in this book, Judith Lorber offered invaluable advice, comments, and encouragement.

Some of the early ideas for this book derive from a plenary talk I gave at an international conference on the changing status of the physicians, a conference organized in Oslo in May 1997 by Olaf Gjerløw Aasland of the Research Institute of the Norwegian Medical Association. That presentation was published later in *Social Science and Medicine* (Riska 2001) and some sections of this book have been adapted from that article. In the fall of 1998, I ran a research seminar on health professions in the Department of Sociology at Åbo Akademi University in Finland. The core participants in this research seminar—Cecilia Benoit, Elina Oinas, Sirpa Wrede—served as a litmus test for the draft versions of the chapters included in this book. From the beginning of the writing, their constructive comments set me on the right track.

A number of other persons have had an important part in enabling me to complete this project. Ann Yrjälä assisted me in conducting interviews with women pathologists. Solveig Bystedt, with her usual patience and kindness, assisted me in preparing the final version of the manuscript. Julia McMurray, Bente Rosenbeck, and Liisa Husu have provided information that has documented some of my main arguments. As a professional editor and longtime friend, Katherine McCracken has provided much-appreciated assistance in detecting the Swedish influence in my English writing. My colleagues and graduate students at my professional base since 1985, the Department of Sociology at Åbo Akademi University, Finland, have offered a most inspiring environment for doing research. Finally, I am indebted to Richard Koffler, the executive director at Aldine de Gruyter, for his interest in my early ideas for this book and for promoting them into publication. I would like to thank Sissy Girard, Mike Sola, and Jan Goldsworthy, who have helped in the production of this book.

A research position as an academy professor granted by the Academy of Finland from 1997 to 2002 offered me an opportunity to embark on the larger comparative research project on women physicians reported in this volume. A subsequent grant (Academy of Finland nos. 53343 and 59221) enabled me to collect data at U.S. university libraries.

                                                                                            Elianne Riska

# 1

## Introduction

Doctor Discontent

Many American doctors are unhappy with the quality of their professional lives. Abundant anecdotal evidence and several surveys identify some of the factors that underlie their discontent. The actions doctors are taking confirm that there is substantial dismay. What are they complaining about, and what are they doing about it? Can a health care system function effectively if a sizeable fraction of its physicians are disgruntled? Are patients well served by unhappy physicians?

Kassirer, "Editorial," *New England Journal of Medicine*

Recent changes in the character of medical work have made the medical profession in many societies concerned about the lack of control over its work. Some of the reactions have been collective and have resulted in strikes or threats of such measures (Burke 1996). Other reactions have taken more individualized expression and are appearing as a growing prevalence of health problems, stress, alcoholism, and suicides among physicians (Stimson 1985; Lindeman, Läärä, Hakko, and Lönnqvist 1996; Arnetz 2001; Firth-Cozens 2001). During the same period that the profession is experiencing a loss of control over the conditions of its work, women have entered the profession in increasing numbers. As new members and with new capacities, will women physicians be able to "humanize" the profession?

The increasing proportion of women in the medical profession has been followed keenly both by conservative and feminist observers during the past three decades. The conservative observers have been mollified by the statistics that show that women physicians remain active members of the profession even after forming a family. But the feminist voices continue to be heard, and for various reasons. One of the early arguments for an increase of women in the medical profession was the quest for equality between the sexes. Liberal feminists demanded that women should have the same educational opportunities as men. Many formal barriers to women's entry into medical schools have been eliminated over recent

1

decades. For example, U.S. medical schools followed affirmative-action policies in the 1970s and 1980s in order to increase the educational opportunities for women.

Subsequently, the focus of criticism has shifted to the skewed career advancement of women within the profession. Statistics both in Europe and in the United States tend to confirm that women work mainly in niches of the health care system or medical specialties characterized by relatively low earnings or prestige. Since the mid-1980s, gender segregation of medical work has become increasingly recognized as a sign of inequality between female and male members of the profession. Furthermore, that women in the profession advance more slowly than men has been alleged to equate with the continuation of discriminatory practices within the profession. Certain structural barriers—such as lack of mentors, collegial support, information, and professional networks that aid career opportunities—have been identified as the mechanisms that hamper women's careers in the profession (Epstein 1970; Lorber 1984, 1993).

In addition to the above structural interpretation of women physicians' position in the medical profession, there is another explanation of the gendered structure of medicine—an essentialist and voluntaristic explanation. According to this view, women harbor essentially different qualities than men (James 1997). This view results in a valorization of women's gender-specific tasks in medicine (e.g., Altekruse and McDermott 1987:85; Ulstad 1993:75). The argument is that the gender division of labor in medical work reflects women's unique female qualities and their own preferences and choices in career decisions rather than discriminatory structures that cluster them in certain niches of medicine. Accordingly, the assumption is that an increase—both numerically and proportionally—of women in the medical profession will in the future radically alter the content of care and the direction of medicine because women can make a special contribution, because of their special gender skills and values. In a health care system with a sizeable proportion of women physicians, patients would encounter more empathic and care-giving physicians. Furthermore, some feminist scholars argue that the sexism inherent in medicine and in the diagnosis and treatment of women patients would disappear as the profession changes from a male-dominated to a more female-dominated one (e.g., Fisher 1995).

These two perspectives address the potential of women physicians in medicine, an issue raised by Lorber (1984, 1985) in her work on women physicians. She predicted that women physicians were likely to be split into two groups: "those who align with other physicians in the fight to maintain professional dominance, and those who align with other female health care workers and consumers in the fight for a health care system with a flatter hierarchy and a holistic and self-care perspective" (Lorber 1985:53). Almost two decades later, there are no major indications of a substantial change in the professional collaboration between women physicians and the nursing profession (e.g., Porter 1992; Gjerberg and Kjølsrød 2001). In fact, the nurses have been actively involved in a professional project of their own, and in a collective mobility project.

As women now constitute almost half and in some countries even the majority of the first-year medical students, the potential of women physicians in the future is an issue that has gained a new prevalence and raised a set of inquiries: Do women physicians represent a potential humanistic and holistic approach to medicine that will head the rest of the profession toward a substantial change in the way medicine is practiced? Or has such a potential been co-opted by a still predominantly male profession that has integrated women as members of the profession but delegated women physicians to marginal and "feminized" niches of medical work where they are ghettoized and mainly pursue traditional female tasks? And to what extent have women physicians at all been able to advance to such positions where they would be able to implement substantial changes in medical practice and medical knowledge?

These questions have to be analyzed from a comparative perspective. Medicine as a social organization is not a universal structure: Health care systems vary in the extent to which physicians work in the private or public sector and in the extent to which they have as a corporate body been able to influence their numbers and the character of their work (e.g., Wilsford 1991; Jones 1991; Moran and Wood 1993; Hafferty and McKinlay 1993; Johnson, Larkin, and Saks 1995). Nor is the gender system a universal one, although some feminist theorists portray it in terms of an all-encompassing patriarchal system (e.g., Walby 1990). Women's social position varies among countries and is related to the country's prevailing gender system. Likewise, the feminist strategies and debates also tend to differ among countries.

This book takes a look at the history and current position of women physicians in three different political and cultural contexts—the United States, the Scandinavian countries—Denmark, Finland, Norway, and Sweden, and Russia/Soviet Union—to illuminate how women's status as professionals has been formed in different settings. In 1950, the proportion of women in the medical profession differed markedly from country to country: In the United States 6 percent of physicians were women, in the Soviet Union 77 percent, in Finland 21 percent, and in the other Scandinavian countries around 10 percent. Today, fifty years later, the Russian figures are almost unchanged, the Scandinavian countries have an almost gender-balanced medical profession, and about one-fourth of U.S. physicians are women.

What are the reasons for these persistent differences, and how far back do they go in the history of medicine in these countries? Have women physicians substantially changed medicine in those countries where they constitute half or a majority of the physicians? Is medicine turning into women's work? These inquiries posed in current literature and public debate have guided the analysis of women physicians' careers and agendas presented in this volume. Broadly characterized, three contexts will serve as analytical tools for understanding the conditions of women physicians and the influence of women physicians: market societies, welfare-state societies, and communist/postcommunist societies.

The title of this book—*Medical Careers and Feminist Agendas: American, Scandinavian, and Russian Women Physicians*—encompasses issues that have been addressed in the research of different disciplines: for example, women's history, sociology of professions, organizational theory, health care policy, social policy, and research on the women's movement. So far, the accumulated knowledge has been descriptive and fragmented. The central argument advanced in this book is that the history of women in medicine provides a lens for the examination of the vast changes that have taken place in medicine. Ever since the entry of women into the medical profession, their presence and agendas have epitomized the major scientific, professional, and organizational transformations of medicine.

In the sociology of professions, major concepts and theories have chiefly been based on a notion of a society as market-oriented, a notion that is not immediately applicable to communist or welfare-state societies, and that does not consider the built-in gender contract in the latter kind of societies. In the Soviet Union, and also in the Scandinavian countries, changes in and the developments of the health care system and health policies have been state endeavors. A majority of the physicians work now, as they have worked in the past, in the public sector.

Much of the research on women physicians has been of a narrow fact-finding nature and consequently detached from the ongoing theoretical discussion within the mainstream of the sociology of professions. Chapter 2 presents an overview of the major theories about professions: the functionalist, the interactionist, the neo-Marxist, the neo-Weberian, and the social-constructionist perspectives. Chapter 2 shows that most of the major sociological theories about professions harbor underlying gendered assumptions. The chapter also looks at theories about work and organizations that have addressed the segregation and hierarchization of work by gender.

The aim of this book is not only to review and to provide an account of women's position in medicine but also to provide an analytical framework that privileges some key sociological issues. The text revolves around three key sociological issues that illuminate this argument: the *numbers, medical practice*, and *feminist agendas* of women physicians. The three issues are addressed in all the chapters but highlighted as central analytical themes in some chapters.

The first key sociological issue—the *number* of women practitioners—relates to women's entry into and later collective mobility in medicine. This issue will be addressed in Chapters 3, 4, and 5.

The pioneering women physicians were a product of and served as catalysts in the fundamental process of social change that signaled the rise of modern society and medicine as an integral part of the modern project. While there were many converging trends in the development in most societies, there were also profound differences. To illustrate these different patterns, Chapters 3, 4, and 5 describe the inroads made by the pioneering women in medicine in the United States, the Scandinavian countries, and Russia in the nineteenth century. The data presented in Chapters 3, 4, and 5 draw on the extensive research done by medical historians. While their approach has focused on individual heroines, my presentation treats these women as a social group and cohort who became part of a collective mobility endeavor of women. In this process, women encountered common barriers but also shared the challenge to move into new activities where women had never worked before.

Chapter 3 looks back at the first entry of women into medicine in the United States and the later practice in medicine in the twentieth century. The chapter provides a summary of the history of the character of medical education available to women during the era of pluralistic medicine (1850–1910) in the United States. In the early 1850s, women began in increasing numbers to enter medical practice in the United States. This early entry was enabled through a separatist strategy—by the establishment of special medical schools for women. Chapter 4 presents an overview of the entry of women into medicine in the Scandinavian countries. Women in the Scandinavian countries entered the profession only in the late 1880s and 1890s, but then immediately through coeducational programs and by earning medical degrees equivalent to those of men. Although the programs were all coeducational from the beginning, the Finnish path was influenced by Finland's ties to Russia, while the other Scandinavian countries followed a somewhat different path. Chapter 5 provides a review of the four phases of medical education—domestic and foreign—available to Russian women before 1917.

While the development in the nineteenth century gives a profile of women physicians as a group, later developments in the proportion and representation of women in the ranks of medicine cannot merely be explained by different early educational policies. In fact, the profile of women's later representation in medicine in the United States and Russia negates such an explanation. For example, in both the United States and Russia women constituted around 6 percent of the medical profession at the turn of the century. While women still constituted 6 percent of the physicians in the United States in 1950, in the Soviet Union as many as

77 percent of the physicians were women. At that time, women constituted 21 percent of the physicians in Finland, a rate equivalent to women's representation in the medical profession in U.S. medicine in the year 2000.

So what has happened in Russian and Finnish medicine during the past fifty years? Can we discern the kind of genuine integration and progressive career advancements that optimistic voices in U.S. medicine are expressing about the future position of women? Is the issue of women's representation in, for example, U.S. medicine today a mere issue of a representational lag? That is, as women enter medicine at the bottom—as students, residents, practicing physicians, and juniors in academic medicine—will their representation gradually level off throughout the system? Or do we find a consistent and permanent pattern of ghettoization of women in medicine, or alternatively a pattern of resegregation in Russian and Scandinavian medicine? Both latter trends confirm a gendering of medical work: Ghettoization suggests that, while men and women have the same job title, they do different jobs—and "gendered niches" of medical practice emerge. Resegregation suggests that an entire occupation or a major occupational specialty is switching from a predominantly male to a predominantly female labor force (Reskin and Roos 1990). In health care, resegregation means that medicine is turning into women's work, and the term "feminization" has been used to illustrate the change from a previously male-dominated occupation to a female-dominated one (Britton 2000). Furthermore, can the past fifty years of history of the careers of women physicians in the Russian and the Finnish health care systems provide some clues about equity between the genders in medicine and about the crumbling of the alleged glass ceiling of medicine? Or does the current high-technology health care industry generate a need at all levels for the kind of holistic and caring skills that women physicians have represented in the past?

Chapters 3, 4, and 5 certainly document that women have advanced in many areas of medicine in all the countries examined here, especially those areas that relate to women's traditional female skills of caring and taking care of children and the elderly. Yet regardless of the proportion of women in medicine—be it in Russia, Scandinavia, or the United States—we find a common pattern of gender segregation. For example, women constitute about 10 percent of the surgeons in U.S. and Scandinavian medicine, while pediatrics seems to be a gender-balanced specialty. But we also find a regressive trend in the hierarchy of medicine: The higher up the echelons of academic and administrative structure of medicine, the lower the representation of women in all the countries examined in this volume.

The representation of women in medicine and career advancement in medicine is a question of gender equality. Chapter 6 looks at the second key sociological issue raised in this book: whether gender really does matter in the *practice of medicine*. As practitioners, are men and women physicians similar or different? In other words, do gender or professional attributes and affiliations matter in the practice of medicine? The chapter presents an overview of two research approaches: the nominal and the embedded. The nominal approach looks at the sex composition of specialties and draws conclusions about the different practice styles of men and women physicians as related to gender. In this approach, gender is treated as a static and individual attribute acquired through sex-role socialization. The embedded approach, on the other hand, does not focus on the individual traits of the physician but rather on gender as a structure and institution. This approach privileges the gendered medical practices and the gendered medical discourses of medicine. This theoretical framework is able to address the divergent practice style of women physicians and to illuminate both their conformity and resistance. The chapter concludes by presenting the typologies suggested by current research on the professional identities and strategies adopted by women physicians. These strategies and identities both confirm and resist the stereotypical gender portrayals of women physicians. The different gendered professional identities indicate that we cannot homogenize women in medicine and that we need to recognize different voices and strategies.

While most of the chapters in this volume address the macrolevel issues of power and professional work in medicine, Chapter 7 analyzes the same issues at the micro level. In focus is women physicians' work in the traditionally male-dominated specialty of pathology. This specialty is, as is surgery, imbued with values and expected capacities of the practitioner that rest on the assumption that the practitioner is a man. This master status of the pathologist is gradually crumbling as pathology increasingly becomes part of the forefront of biomedicine, i.e., medicine done through microscopy, exemplified by cancer research, medical genetics, and molecular biology. Women physicians working as pathologists are in many respects pioneers. Pathology is a consulting specialty: It provides expert opinions to other physicians on the health of their patient. Pathologists do not meet patients; instead a decontexualized fragment of the body—the tissue sample—serves as the representation of the body. The work requires visual skills: a way of seeing and reading the body through the tissue. This visual skill can in Foucault's (1975) terms be called the pathological or the microscopic gaze (Atkinson 1995). Chapter 7 describes how women physicians have had to challenge the master status of the pathologist—a medical man who does autopsies—and construct their craft skills in gendered terms. It shows that the internal differentiation by gender is constructed by means of gender casting and gender inclusion, whereby women pathologists see themselves assigned certain gender-specific skills and tasks.

Chapter 8 addresses the third key sociological issue, which concerns the *feminist agenda* that women physicians originally set for themselves and how this issue has been addressed in the later developments of medicine. Most of the pioneering women physicians were part of the contemporary women's movement at the turn of the century, and worked for a women's health agenda as a way of improving women's position in society, as is shown in Chapters 3, 4, and 5. Later, as women physicians were integrated into mainstream medicine, their ability to work for and commitments to women's causes began to fade. The separatist and integrationist strategies for women's practice in medicine have been a major marker between the policies waged by women's groups in various countries, as most chapters in this book will show. At issue has been how women can change medicine: Can they best change it from within or from without?

In the 1970s, with the second wave of the women's movement, women's health returned as an issue in most Western societies. But how did women physicians relate to the challenge from the outside by lay-women health advocates? A women's health movement emerged in the 1970s, for example, in the United States, Great Britain, and Australia. These movements were not headed by women physicians but by lay-women who reclaimed the right of women to define their health needs in their own terms and to have control over their bodies and their treatment. The concrete outcome of the movement was the emergence of feminist women's health centers, most of which represented a critical stance toward mainstream medicine, regardless of the gender of the physician.

Chapter 8 provides a case study of the women's health movement in the United States and looks at the evolution of three phases that capture how and by whom women's health has been advocated over the past thirty years: by laywomen in the 1970s, by commercialized ventures in the 1980s, and by professional advocates in the 1990s. The chapter reviews how women's health issues have been integrated into the health care provided by the welfare state in the Scandinavian countries. A key question is whether this has meant that women's health has been co-opted by the medical profession and whether the women's health movement is missing from feminism in the Scandinavian countries.

The concluding Chapter 9 pulls together the common themes of the preceding chapters and suggests a way forward. It returns to the three key sociological issues—numbers, medical practice, and feminist agendas—and readdresses them in the light of the material presented in the individual chapters and against the backdrop of current mainstream sociological theory of professions. The chapter addresses three concerns that the material in this book has covered. First, what theories best explain the data on women physicians' careers? Second, what strategies seem to have the best payoff for women's advancement in medicine? Third, what kind of changes have women physicians made and what contributions are women physicians likely to make in the future?

# 2

# Sociological Theories about
# Medical Work and Gender

Under what circumstances, if ever, is the "hen doctor" simply a doctor? And who are the first to accept her as such—her colleagues or her patients? Will the growth of a separate superstructure over each of the segregated bottom groups of our society tend to perpetuate indefinitely the racial and ethnic division already existing, or will these superstructures lose their identity in the general organization of society? These are the larger questions.

—Everett C. Hughes

## MAJOR THEORETICAL PERSPECTIVES
## ON MEDICAL WORK

Over the past thirty years women have in increasing numbers entered areas in working-life—medicine, law, engineering, science, management—considered previously to require the qualities of men. As women continue to increase in these previously male-dominated areas of work, two questions have been raised: Do women and men differ in their approach to work? Why are there still so few women in top positions of the organizations that the work entails? (See, e.g., Billing and Alvesson 1989:63.) The first question addresses the issue of segregation of work, while the other concerns the hierarchization of work. The two issues are currently debated within three separate scholarly communities: the sociology of professions, organizational theory, and feminist theory. The common theme addressed by these three theoretical traditions is the character of and reasons for social differentiation in society, but the scholarship in each tradition has been pursued in relative isolation from the others.

The three theoretical traditions address the issue of social differentiation in different ways. The theories about professions have focused on why and how professions differ from occupations in order to explain the special power exerted by professions. Organizational theories have focused on structural determinants and cultural factors as alternative explanations of organizational behavior. Feminist theories have raised the issue of gender differences: some from the point of view of inequality between men and women, and others as a special value and contribution that women may bring to the way society is organized. The issue of gender has not to the same extent been problematized in the sociology of professions as it has in organizational theory. While women and management is a subject that has been extensively covered in organizational research during the past twenty years, the same cannot be said about the issue of gender in the sociology of professions. Gender seems to be both an underresearched and undertheorized issue in theories about professions.

The following sections will give an overview of the major theories debated in the three theoretical traditions—sociology of professions, organizational theory, and feminist theory—concerning women's presumed impact on the way work is done. The sections on the sociology of professions and organizational theory also discuss how the different theoretical perspectives address segregation and hierarchization of work by gender.

## GENDER AND THEORIES ON PROFESSIONS

Until the mid-1980s, mainstream theories in the sociology of professions were for the most part gender blind or based on the assumption that medical work was done by men. In both cases, professions were tacitly assumed to be composed of men, and the professional traits and behaviors were generally portrayed in masculine terms. Both views made women physicians invisible members of the profession. As women have entered professions (medicine in particular) in greater numbers, new questions about the character of professions and of women's impact have been raised. Some have argued that professions are intrinsically male-gendered while others have proposed that women can bring into professions—as in the case of medicine and management—new values that will change the practice style of the profession as a whole.

This section looks at current theories in the sociology of professions from a gender perspective, specifically examining the kind of views, if any, they may have about the role of gender in the organization of work within the profession. Currently five major theoretical perspectives can be identified in the debate about the character of the medical profession: (1) the functionalist, (2) the interactionist, (3) the neo-Marxist, (4) the neo-Weberian, and (5) the social constructionist. Figure 2.1 summarizes the views that these perspectives have on three issues: the underlying structure of professions, the major focus of analysis of the perspective, and the underlying assumptions about the role of gender in the organization of work.

| Perspective | Underlying structure | Focus of analysis | Gender aspects of the profession |
|---|---|---|---|
| Functionalist: | | | |
| Parsons | Normative consensus (pattern variables) | Professional role of physicians | Professional socialization and professional behavior are gender-neutral per definition |
| Interactionist: | | | |
| Hughes | Social drama of work | Occupational work and culture | Master status is male gendered |
| Freidson | Professional knowledge | Medical work | Professional dominance of (male) physicians |
| Neo-Weberian | Modern society and rationalization | Gendered organization of health care | Gendered professional projects |
| Neo-Marxist: | | | |
| Navarro | | Corporate and bureaucratic structure of health care | Women physicians are class allies with medical men |
| McKinlay | Capitalist economy | | Proletarianized status of women physicians |
| Postmodern/social constructionist | Social practices and discourses | Medical and lay discourses | Gendered character of social practices and discourses |

*Figure 2.1.* Theoretical perspectives on the medical profession and underlying assumptions about gender.

Among these perspectives, the representatives of the neo-Marxist, the neo-Weberian, and the social-constructionist perspective have explicitly addressed the gender dimension of the medical profession. Although the functionalist perspective has a gender-neutral outlook on professions, it has been enormously influential because of one of its strands: socialization theory. In the past, socialization theory has, especially in U.S. sociology, been the perspective most frequently used to explain social differentiation in society (Ferree and Hall 1996).

According to the *functionalist perspective* on professions, the role of physician is an institutionalized social role, the task of which is the regulation of the kind of deviance interpreted as based on illness. The professions constitute a prototype that captures the kind of social relationships that have emerged in modern society. The normative pattern, guiding the professions in modern society, is achievement, universalism, functional specificity, affective neutrality, and collectivity orientation (Parsons 1951: 454). Hence, professions constitute a special structure within the wider society, and the norms guiding the behavior of the professional are quite different from those prevailing in the private sphere, notably family and kinship (Parsons 1949:193). For Parsons, the two structures exist in "relative insulation" from each other so that the value pattern guiding one area is supposed not to carry over to the other, even if the same concrete individuals inhabit both spheres (ibid.:197). For Parsons, then, the particularistic orientation of any ascribed status—such as gender or race—would not interfere with the behavior of the same person occupying a professional role. The argument is that a woman physician is above all a physician. Her achieved status and the concomitant professional identity and behavior will guide her own interaction as well as that of her colleagues and patients.[1]

The functionalist perspective is based on a view of normative consensus. The institutionalized roles of the physician and the sick person—the so-called sick role—contain certain expectations as well as obligations concerning expected behavior related to the role. The role of the physician is acquired through a period of professional socialization where both the technical knowledge and the norms guiding professional behavior are taught. The views about the character of this socialization process were covered in a classic, *The Student Physician* (Merton, Reader, and Kendall 1957), that was based on a functionalist perspective. As the study showed, medical students are acquiring an attitude of "detached concern" and being trained for situations characterized by uncertainty. These attitudes and norms concerning professional conduct are adopted as part of the professional role of and professional career as a physician. As Lorber (1975:85) has pointed out, this classic did not mention gender at all. Later reviews have pointed to the assumption of the functionalist perspective: professional socialization overrules the previous impact of primary socialization, such as gender socialization (Levinson 1967; Martin, Arnold, and Parker 1988).

The *interactionist perspective* on medical work has its earliest representative in a study on the professional socialization of medical students by a group of sociologists at the University of Chicago (Becker, Geer, Hughes, and Strauss 1961), and in Everett Hughes's (1958) collection of essays *Men and Their Work*. For Hughes, the focus of a study of any kind of occupation is the "social drama of work" (ibid.:53). In his view, most occupations bring together people in definable roles and the content of work and status are defined in their interaction. An occupation is not a priori by means of its expertise and knowledge a profession but a social status that is socially constructed (ibid.:44–45). According to Hughes, the aim of the study of the work of occupations and professions should therefore be "to *penetrate more deeply* into the personal and social drama of work, to understand the social and social-psychological arrangements and devices by which men make their work tolerable, or even glorious to themselves and others" (ibid.:48).

Although Hughes uses masculine terms for the person doing the physician's work, and female terms for nurses, he raises the issue of the status incongruences of those members of the profession who do not have the expected status traits. He introduces the term *master status* for the formal status. This formal status has auxiliary traits—for example, a woman and a black physician deviate from the "expected [white, male] type." Hughes illustrates his argument by pointing to the sixteen likely medical encounters that would result if the physician and the patient inhabited any of two other statuses—race (black or white) and gender (female or male) (ibid.:107).

The internal control system within the profession, which Hughes calls "the colleague-group," strives to maintain homogeneity to protect the "secrets" and the work of the profession. As Hughes notes: "The colleague-group is ideally a brotherhood; to have within it people who cannot, given one's other attitudes, be accepted as brothers is very uncomfortable" (ibid.:112; 1945:355).

The inclusionary device is "social segregation," and Hughes foresees the gender-segregated pattern of medical practice to appear fifty years later: "Women physicians may find a place in those specialties of which women and children have need" (1958:113). Another solution, which he also views as a kind of segregation and isolation, "is that of putting the new people in the library or laboratory, where they get the prestige of research but are out of the way of patients and the public" (ibid.:114). These are the tasks that later literature has called "gender-based integration" and "occupational niches" (Reskin and Roos 1990:49) for women, which are visible in the statistics in the form of gender segregation of jobs (men work with men and women with women) and the gender stratification of organizational hierarchies (the top of the pyramid is almost all men) (Lorber 1998:21).

From a gender perspective, Hughes's view of the medical profession is different from his contemporaries' in many ways. First, although he, like them, uses male terms for the primary holder of membership in the professions, he raises the issue of gender as a status. In today's words, Hughes argues that the master status of the medical profession is male gendered. Second, he conceptualizes gender explicitly as a status and not as a role, as Parsons does, and manages in that way to contextualize gender as a social category related to larger social structures. Third, as indicated in the quotation in the very beginning of this chapter, Hughes raises the larger question of the assimilation or perpetuation of the marginal status and identity of women as a group at various levels in the organization of society. The question is raised in some later works by, for example, Reskin and Roos (1990:71) about the possible routes that occupational desegregation can take: genuine integration, ghettoization, and resegregation.

Working within the interactionist tradition is another sociologist, Erving Goffman, whose work is seldom considered part of the sociology of professions. Goffman's work on the asylum focuses on the power and control of the medical profession and the routine work of health care personnel. Like Hughes, Goffman (1961:325–26) perceives professions not as intrinsically distinct from occupations but rather as a particular type of personal-service occupation based on expertise. For Goffman, an expert provides a special type of "tinkering service": "The ideals underlying expert servicing in our society are rooted in the case where the server has a complex physical system to repair, construct, or tinker with—the system here being the client's personal object or possession." Tinkering services contain a series of distinct phases, which constitute the "repair cycle" (ibid.:330). The medical version of the tinkering-services model confronts, however, a major problem—the body. It is a possession of the served that cannot be left under the care of the server while the client goes about his or her other business. A large part of the medical encounter contains, therefore, "non-person treatment" or ways of handling the patient/the body as "a possession someone has left behind" (ibid.:341). Furthermore, the verbal part of the server's exchange contains three components: a technical part that contains the relevant repair information, a contractual part that specifies the terms of the repair task, and the sociable part that involves courtesies, civilities, and signs of deference (ibid.:328–29).

During the past decade, the dilemma of the presence of the body in medical encounters and the physician's preference for focusing on the technical part while being oblivious to the social part of the verbal exchange has been the focus of a whole new genre of research. Based on the interactionist framework, several studies have examined the interaction between clients and health care experts. A new method—conversational analysis—has been one of the outcomes of this research (Silverman 1987; Atkinson and Heritage 1984; Psathas 1995; Peräkylä 1995, 1997).

Goffman's work on the expert's role is gender-blind but is certainly amenable to an analysis that emphasizes the gendered criteria in the presentation of self and in the interaction between the expert and the client. An effort to introduce such a view into the analysis of medical work has been done by West (1993), who has used the concept "doing gender" as an analytical tool to highlight the gender aspect of physicians' work.

A third representative of the interactionist approach is Freidson and his work on the U.S. medical profession. The *professional dominance perspective*, introduced by Freidson (1970, 1984, 1985), is a gender-blind theory.[2] Freidson does not identify gender as one of the organizing principles in professional dominance asserted by or in his views on the emerging internal differentiation of the medical profession. Freidson (1984, 1985) views the new internal differentiation of the profession as a way of accommodating itself to the ongoing corporatization and rationalization of medicine. The three divisions are the physicians involved in medical education and research, the physicians having administrative positions in practice organizations, and the rank-and-file physicians (Freidson 1985:30). This is Freidson's "restratification" thesis. The divisions within medicine are perceived by function, both horizontally and vertically, but these divisions are not perceived as overlapping with gender (ibid.).

It would, however, have been possible to include gender in the accommodation argument of the restratification thesis. A gender perspective would have implied an identification of women physicians as increasingly occupying the rank-and-file positions with men maintaining the positions that protect the boundaries of the profession—that is, the knowledge and the administrative elite of the profession. But, as critics have suggested, Freidson focuses mainly on the internal organization of medical work. The argument about the restratification of the medical profession is not related to views on how society is otherwise organized by gender, race, or class. This has led Coburn (1992) to suggest that Freidson's work on the medical profession lacks a systematic theory of society.

By contrast, the *neo-Marxist perspective* relates the power of the profession to the larger underlying economic and political organization of society. According to the neo-Marxist perspective on professions, capitalist society determines the superstructure, of which the social organization of health care, the professions, and medicine as a science are but parts. As its most ardent representative suggests: "The same economic and political forces that determine the class structure of the United States also determine the nature and the functions of the U.S. health sector" (Navarro 1975:90). The argument here is that the same hierarchy is found in the health sector as in the rest of the capitalist economy. "At the top we find the physicians," and "the majority of persons in this group are white and male, besides being upper middle-class" (ibid.:70). Subordinated to this group at the top are the paraprofessionals, and "this group is primarily female and is part of the lower-income" (ibid.:90). This female labor force is in focus in an essay entitled "The labor force: women as producers of services in the health sector of the United States" (Navarro 1976:170–79), which still over two decades later remains one of the few comprehensive reviews written on the topic. The argument presented is that "to understand the present situation of women as producers in the health sector, we must also understand the distribution of political and economic power in the world of men" (ibid.:170). Gender discrimination in the health sector is interpreted as related to the social and economic role of the family, in which the man is the breadwinner and women are treated only as a reserve army of workers in the labor force (ibid.:174–75). Any change of women's situation in the health labor force is seen as related to "the patterns of control of that sector" and "a change in the sex and class composition and the system of governance of the agencies in the health sector and its institutions" (ibid.:176). Navarro is clearly more interested in the plight of working-class women of the health labor force than the dominant "focus on the problems faced by professional women" (ibid.:170). Nor is he very optimistic about the potential for change that female physicians may represent and predicts that their class loyalties are far stronger than their gender loyalties, with the result that they will not ally with the female-dominated "working class" of health service workers in the health labor force (ibid.:178).

All the perspectives above perceive the medical profession as united, powerful, and male-dominated. The prophecy of a gradual loss of the power of the medical profession is attributed to two other sociologists, Marie Haug (1975) and John McKinlay (McKinlay and Arches 1985; McKinlay and Stoeckle 1988), who have advanced the *deprofessionalization* and *proletarianization* theses, respectively. The theoretical framework of the two is, however, different. Haug's underlying theory of society is a postindustrial one, while McKinlay and his colleagues use a Marxist framework. The term postindustrial society implies a society headed by experts, but Haug challenges the orthodox postindustrial society theory that assigns the professional elite power and control over society. According to her, the knowledge monopoly of the medical profession is challenged both by various female health professionals and by clients who have increasing access to medical knowledge through the information industry. The prophecy of Haug is that the prerogatives of the medical profession will wither away because "professions are rapidly losing their control over their knowledge domain as a result of inroads from computerization, new occupations in the division of labor, and increasing public and client sophistication" (1975:211).

McKinlay and his colleagues adopt a neo-Marxist perspective: Medicine is viewed as being taken over by capital-intensive and large corporations, a development that will result in physicians working increasingly as salaried employees of such organizations. The term "proletarianization" of physicians denotes a process that will gradually result in the loss of the traditional power of the profession. The assumption is that all physicians will lose professional power and autonomy, since the corporatization of medicine is perceived as an ongoing universal process. This neo-Marxist view differs from that of Freidson, who suggests that the emergence of different segments of the profession—or functions, as he calls them—is the very stronghold of the profession in its endeavor to maintain professional dominance. As noted above, Freidson does not recognize the gendered elements in the emerging internal differentiation.

McKinlay recognizes, however, that "the division of labor in health care is increasingly stratified by age and gender, with female and younger doctors disproportionately in salaried positions" (McKinlay and Stoeckle 1988:195). This feature of medicine is in later works called the rise of bureaucratic medicine (McKinlay and Marceau 1998). The salaried position of women physicians can in strictly Marxist terms be interpreted as wage labor and hence as "proletarianized" work. So, the rise of wage labor and large bureaucracies creates a group of professionals who lack control over their work. This subordinated status has by many been equated with the kind of status women tend to occupy in working life. Hence, the term "feminization" of work has not only implied a rise in the number of female members of a previously male-dominated profession but also contains a notion of low status and little control over work associated with the female workers in the labor force at large (e.g., Reskin and Roos 1990; Britton 2000). Others have argued, however, that the increasing bureaucratization of medical practice has implied regular work hours and therefore given women and young physicians increased control over their work and thereby given more time for family. In addition, bureaucratized medicine provides women and young physicians an alternative to the financial risks and capital investment involved in entrepreneurial self-employment (Carpenter 1977:204; Reskin and McBrier 2000).

Inherent in the proletarianization thesis is, however, an implicit recognition of a dual labor market for physicians: one for women and younger physicians and another for the older male physicians still clinging to the privileges of professional autonomy. Women are said to be absorbed by the labor market dominated by large corporations while the male physicians remain in the labor market characterized by a cottage-industry type of market conditions. In the case of physicians, contrary to orthodox dual-labor-market theory, the capital-intensive primary market of salaried physicians is not related to good pay and career advancement but to increasing proletarianization, while the men's entrepreneurial market is associated with a sense of autonomy of the profession and high economic status.

Reskin and Roos (1990:308–9) have examined the segregation of labor markets from a gender perspective and introduced an interpretation they call the *queueing perspective*. There are two types of queueing processes: labor queues that order groups of workers according to their attractiveness to employers, and job queues that rank jobs according to their attractiveness to workers. Their own study of long-term developments in the U.S. labor market showed four conditions that "feminized" occupations: occupational growth changed the shape of job queues, workers reordered jobs in some queues in response to changing relative rewards, employers' gender preference adapted to attitudinal change in society, and women's share of labor queues for male occupations expanded.

The queueing perspective highlights the structural properties of labor markets and the collective character of gender segregation and in this way redirects the attention from a narrow focus on the characteristics of female workers (ibid.:308). It also considers noneconomic factors, e.g., attitudes, ideology, in the rankings performed by workers and employers. Britton calls this perspective on work and organizations "the nominal approach" (2000:424). She draws a distinction between the sex composition and gender-typing of an organization or occupation.

The former indicates the numerical representation of one gender in, for example, an occupation, whereas the latter reflects the ranking of gender in society. As Epstein in her pioneering work in this field suggested, sex-typing reflects sex-ranking: "Men rank first in the ranking of the sexes and they get the first ranking-jobs" (1970:162).

According to the *neo-Weberian perspective*, professions are occupational groups that operate in the marketplace and have been successful in demarcating the domain of their work as their exclusionary right (Larson 1977; Parkin 1979). The neo-Weberian approach to the professions emerged as a reaction to the functionalist and traits perspective on professions (Saks 1983). In focus are the characteristics of medical work and the actions of the occupational group striving for a professional status and defending it through the strategy of closure. Witz (1992) has added a feminist perspective in her neo-Weberian analysis of the power of the medical profession, nurses, and midwives in the United Kingdom and suggests that professions have always been gendered projects—i.e., the agents are either men or women. For example, Witz argues that, following the Medical Registration Act of 1858 in Great Britain, "medical men used gendered exclusionary strategies to maintain a male monopoly of registered medical practice" (ibid.:6).

Witz points to four strategies of occupational closure. The *exclusionary* strategies consist of intra-occupational control over internal affairs and allows a collegial control over the members. The *demarcationary* strategies entail interoccupational control over the affairs of related or adjacent occupations in the division of labor (ibid.:44). *Inclusionary* strategies may be used by subordinated groups who seek entry into a group from which they have been excluded. And *dual-closure* strategies are employed by subordinated groups that challenge the profession's intra-occupational control while they at the same time consolidate their own position by means of exclusion (see also Nettleton 1995:200). In this regard, Witz portrays biomedicine as a male professional project that has subjugated all other female health occupations in the emerging male-dominated hierarchy of medical work. According to Witz, in the medical profession the exclusionary strategy has had a gendered form. On the one hand, the medical profession has exerted gendered collectivist criteria of exclusion vis-á-vis women while, on the other hand, it has used gendered individualist criteria of inclusion vis-á-vis men. Here the implicit argument is that medicine will be a high-status profession as long as it remains a male professional project.

The *social-constructionist approach* treats medicine as both historically and culturally located.

More recently the work of Foucault (1975; Turner 1997; Armstrong 1983, 1995, 1997) has inspired sociologists to analyze the themes of power and the social control aspect of medicine from a constructionist perspective. For Foucault, power is a relationship that is typically disguised through a social system, and its specific practices operate at several levels. The disciplinary practices are perceived as regimes that produce institutions, individuals, and cultural arrangements (Turner 1997; Armstrong 1983, 1997). In the medical profession, power and knowledge are exerted through the medical gaze that is a frame through which diseases are identified and constructed into distinct categories and bestowed on the body. But medical knowledge is not the sole prerogative of the medical profession, since only by means of a cultural system—be it the orthodox medical discourse or the lay discourse of the body—can the body be understood, experienced, and acted upon.

Atkinson (1995), however, challenges the way that biomedicine or the so-called orthodox medical discourse has been conceptualized in sociological and anthropological research as one unitary discourse. Instead of what Mishler (1984) and the genre of studies on conversation analysis in medical encounters have done, constructing a dichotomy between the "voice of medicine" and the "voice of the lifeworld," Atkinson asks for an analysis of the "voices of medicine." He suggests that the medical profession is divided into different segments and, furthermore, not all of them are involved in patient care.

The implicit assumption in much of the work on the profession has been that the social is to be found with the patient. In previous research of physicians' work, the focus has been the patient-physician interaction where the culture of illness and the asymmetrical power relation between the physician and the patient have constituted the social aspects of medicine. In this way, medical work itself has been left underexplored (Strauss, Fagerhaugh, Suczek, and Wiener 1985:xi; Atkinson 1995:34). In today's complex division of labor in medical institutions, medical work is conducted in "variegated workshops" (Strauss et al. 1985:6) involving various types of health professionals but also done as a product of a physician-to-physician interaction. The latter work has been referred to as *medical knowledge production*—knowledge produced and reproduced through occupational talk about what has been read as the signs of the body. Atkinson's (1995) own study concerned the work of hematologists, and he shows that the production of expert knowledge is a process of collegial, occupational talk to confirm "biomedical reality" and to initiate students to the field. The narrative productions of the physicians are a distinct rhetoric of medical talk that constructs and confirms medical knowledge. But this knowledge production has a gendered character, which Atkinson does not bring up but which will be shown in Chapter 7 of this volume. This chapter provides a microsociological account of the occupational talk and craft skills associated with women pathologists.

The Foucauldian theory of the power surrounding medicine has in the 1990s attracted those who have wanted to understand changes taking place in the governance of health care. Many feminists have found Foucault's gender-neutral theory of power problematic despite the potential inherent in the concepts of medical discourse and regimes. Hence, a separate feminist theory on the construction of the female body has emerged, addressing the lack of gender in previous social-constructionist approaches (e.g., Bordo 1993; Butler 1993; Lorber 1996, 1997; Davis 1995; Witz 2000). According to feminist proponents of the social-constructionist approach, medicine is a discursive strategy waged by the male-dominated profession. As Davies (1996:673) suggests, the professions constitute a system of gendered relations, and what contemporary professions profess is masculine gender. The merit of the feminist approach is that it focuses on women's status in the medical profession (and also in nursing) and points to the need to unravel the social and cultural practices that define and confirm women's work in the division of labor in health care. On the other hand, this approach can result in a narrow, cultural interpretation of the organization of medical work. More important, it may easily result in the neglect of class and race divisions within medical work (Carpenter 1993). It can also lead to a disregard of the external and powerful influences that, for example, the state and large corporate enterprises exert on health care and on the medical profession.

## SOCIOLOGICAL EXPLANATIONS OF THE GENDERED CHARACTER OF MEDICAL WORK

Recent restructuring of health care systems and its effects on women's career opportunities in medicine have resulted in a call for a shift in analysis from that of the single profession of medicine and its internal structure to the larger social organization of medicine and its division of labor. Such an approach highlights the relationship between gender and the structure of health care as an organization.

In the study of the relationship between gender and organizations, there are three main theoretical perspectives or approaches: the contingent, the embedded, and the essentialist (Halford, Savage, and Witz 1997:1). The *contingent approach* represents a view that assumes that current organizations are fundamentally gender neutral and that their gendered character is the contingent outcome of specific historical circumstances and not an intrinsic feature of bureaucratic organizations (ibid.:6). The *embedded approach* conceptualizes any organization as a socially situated practice and sees gender as embedded in any organization of society (ibid.:13–15; Acker 1990, 1992; Rantalaiho and Heiskanen 1997; Britton 2000). The *essentialist approach* suggests that an organization reflects the inherent characteristics of its dominant occupants, so that, for example, a bureaucratic organization is inherently a masculine form of organizing work (Halford et al. 1997:10).

### The Contingent Approach

The foregoing three approaches are also represented in the theoretical perspectives on professions and management. The contingent approach is advanced by scholars who have proposed a gender-neutral view of professions and those who have viewed the male-dominated character of professions as a historical remnant and cultural lag that will gradually be corrected as women enter higher education in greater numbers and also aspire to higher academic degrees and positions in the profession. The lag interpretation is, for example, expressed in the normative barriers approach and the structural barriers approach to gender inequality (Fiorentine and Cole 1992).

The *normative barriers approach* is the most frequently cited explanation of gender inequality and underrepresentation of women in high status and executive positions in the professions. This perspective suggests that there are normative barriers hampering women's advancement as individuals and as a group in the labor market and in occupations and professions (Ferree and Hall 1996). This theory focuses on socialization processes shaping gender traits and so-called sex or gender roles. It is assumed that women have been socialized in ways that stress conformity to traditional female values—the home, family, and children as the primary concern for women. Even if women decide to enter higher education and working life, they will choose those areas where the same family-oriented values and tasks are valorized. There allegedly are normative barriers to breaking the traditional, gender-related normative expectations and values related to women's traditional position in the family and society.

Socialization theory has also been used to explain recent changes in the gender composition of professions such as medicine and law. The argument has been that changes in gender socialization and more liberal norms about tasks that can be done by men and women constitute the primary reason for the rise in the proportion of women in previously male-dominated professions. Young women are currently offered more affirmative and achievement-oriented role models and feel more free to choose among different career options.

This explanation does not consider elimination of barriers previously erected and the changes in the labor market and the internal structure of the profession that have opened up new opportunity structures for women (Ferree and Hall 1996:940). For example, the restructuring of health care systems that has been going on in most Western societies has created new career opportunities for women and new jobs in niches of medicine (Williams 1999). This development has not affected men physicians, who remain in the traditional and prestigious areas of medicine, like surgery and private practice. In this regard, socialization theory reduces the unequal location of men and women within the profession to gender socialization and individual career choices. In this way, gender itself is conceptualized as a static trait while the values and norms are seen as those that are changing.

As applied to the medical profession, socialization theory has two strands: one that explains the existence of gender differences, and another that explains the lack of gender differences. The first one points to the way that young people are socialized into traditional gender roles, how gender-related preferences explain career choices, and how the acquisition of female gender traits impedes advancement within the profession. It is argued, for example, that women lack the kind of traits needed for achievement within professions that are highly competitive. Such a *deficiency focus* explains women's location in the division of labor within medicine as a product of characteristics shared by women—for example, women's lack of the competitive and instrumental orientation required in some areas of medicine, such as research and surgery. Similarly, the *asset focus* explains women's work in certain specialties as related to their special female skills. For example, the overrepresentation of women physicians in specialties catering to children and the elderly has been perceived as related to women's special affinity to and contribution in caring work in society.

There is also another version of socialization theory, in which the professional role of physicians is viewed as gender neutral since both female and male medical students are socialized in essentially the same way. It is also argued that the content and demands of scientific medicine give little space for gender-socialized traits (see, e.g., Levinson 1967; Martin et al. 1988). Hence, professional socialization is seen as a process that overrules the effects of gender socialization. As a consequence, any incumbent in a physician role will display gender-neutral professional behavior. This perspective follows the view of professional socialization and professional behavior introduced in Parsons's work (1949, 1951; see also Merton et al. 1957).

This latter version of the socialization perspective has at least two shortcomings. First, it makes gender invisible although the gender-neutral patterns and behaviors observed are often based on male premises and the gendered structures of medicine. Second, it portrays the profession as a homogeneous and united body and assumes that any changes will affect its members equally.

The second major explanation of the underrepresentation of women in high-status professional and executive positions is represented by the *structural barriers approach*. This approach views the structural barriers of an organization as the major reason for women's lack of advancement or of their slow advancement in the career pattern of an organization or within a profession. Classics promoting this perspective are the works by Cynthia Fuchs Epstein (1970) and Rosabeth Moss Kanter (1977).

The concept of gatekeeping has been introduced to explain how women are kept from getting to the top of organizations or professions dominated by men. While the doors to most professional careers are today open to women, more subtle mechanisms are at work, such as networking and access to mentors. This structural mechanism is the protègè and mentor system suggested by Epstein (1970). The mentor is a senior colleague who provides the informal professional socialization in the secrets of professional conduct and knowledge. According to Epstein's explanation, women medical students are not to the same extent as their male fellow students connected to a mentor and buddy system that would provide them with the kind of informal socialization and information channels generally available to men. Lorber (1984:6–8) has pointed to the peer-regulation mechanism of medicine, which assigns the gatekeepers the task of sorting out the members of the profession. The gatekeepers in medicine tend to be men, and Lorber (1993:63) argues in her later work that "there is a 'glass ceiling' on women physicians' upward mobility" within the medical profession that makes the top positions male-dominated. This is the exclusionary strategy that Hughes (1958:112) identified as being pursued by the "colleague-group" within the profession.

The concept of the glass ceiling has been recently the subject of debate in U.S. sociology (e.g., Alessio and Andrzejewski 2000; Baxter and Wright 2000; Ferree and Purkayastha 2000). At issue has been whether the glass ceiling is a generic concept, or one that describes a specific pattern of disadvantage that women encounter at a certain level in an organizational hierarchy, or one that denotes the cumulative effects of constant promotion differentials at all levels. As applied to medicine, the interpretation of the glass ceiling as a matter of cumulative effects seems best to describe women physicians' careers (see Chapters 3 and 4).

Kanter (1977) focused on organizational behavior related to the person's position in the organization and more specifically to the opportunity structure in the organization. Some positions provide opportunities for a career, while other positions are dead-end jobs. Although men tend to occupy the former and women the latter, Kanter argues that there is nothing intrinsically male or female about these kinds of jobs, but the behavior, regardless of gender, is shaped by the position and opportunity structure in the organization. Another argument of the hypothesis is that the proportional representation of a social category in the organization will influence the behavior and power of that group in the leadership of the organization. For example, women tend to constitute tokens in management positions as long as they remain a small minority, but when their proportion increases to more than about 35 percent, their token status will change. Kanter assumes that when an organization becomes more gender-balanced, women will begin to have real influence in the organization. This is the so-called Kanter hypothesis about behavior in organizations. To this sociology-of-numbers argument, the critics have suggested that the numbers are not the crucial fact—rather, the male-gendered character of organizations is (Zimmer 1988; Blum and Smith 1988; Acker 1990, 1992; Williams 1992; Britton 2000).

The contingent and the structural approaches to the gender segregation of work tend to conceal the underlying gendered structure of organizations or professions. The contingent approach presents the current unequal distribution of men and women in various areas and ranks of medicine as the

result of a temporary representational lag. The assumption is that as women embark on their career, their majority at the bottom of the career ranks
will filter through the various fields and hierarchies of medicine. This slow
but steady flow of women upwards in the career ranks of medicine will create not only a gender-balanced but even a female-dominated profession
within the near future. This theory of the temporary representational lag
of women physicians in medicine is frequently espoused by representatives of medicine.

The structural approach recognizes the structural barriers for women's
advancement but sees these barriers mainly as practical problems. Once
they are identified and acted upon, women and men will be treated
equally in the organization. This is a view often held by liberal feminists.
Yet such a perspective generally ignores that individuals act in gendered
institutions and that the gender of institutions influences the behavior of
men and women in them regardless of their gender identities (Acker 1992;
Kimmel 2000).

## The Embedded Approach

The embedded approach questions the gender neutrality of organizations or professions. The argument is that organizations and professions
are linked to gender as an institution in society. The exponents of this view
argue that a certain representation of gender is prevalent in Western societies: a binary notion. The binary notion of gender entails not only that
there are merely two gender categories—men and women—but also that
the two categories are of unequal worth (Lorber 1994:35; 2000b). This
social construction of gender creates a gender system with a built-in gender inequality.

The gender system operates at two levels: through gendered processes
and through gendered practices. The term "gendered processes" denotes
the ongoing production of hierarchies of social difference by gender. At the
macro level such processes produce rankings of jobs that some have called
"gender queueing" (Reskin and Roos 1990) and others "sex-typing"
(Epstein 1970). Sex-typing of an occupation is a phenomenon equivalent to
Hughes's concept of "master status." As shown previously in this chapter,
Hughes called attention to what today would be called the embodied status of occupations—certain positions are associated with the expected
gender traits and rankings of other statuses. More recently the embodied
master status and sex-typing of physicians who work, for example, in specialties like general practice and surgery (Hinze 1999; Cassell 2000) have
been documented (see Chapter 6).

The embedded approach to professions has been used in this book as
the major theoretical framework for understanding the social construction

of skills and jurisdictions of physicians working in certain specialties of medicine.

## The Essentialist Approach

The essentialist approach suggests that professions are tied to the specific culture of the two genders. There are those who focus on the masculine culture and there are others who privilege the female. Those who identify professions as a patriarchal culture argue that professions constitute an inherently masculine way of organizing work. The radical feminist view falls within this way of defining the traits of professions. For example, Ehrenreich and English (1973, 1978) give such an account in their classic study on the rise of the male-dominated medical profession. The backdrop of the current male-dominated medical profession is interpreted in patriarchal terms: "It was an active *takeover* by male professionals" (Ehrenreich and English 1973:4). Before this male takeover, women worked as "wise women" representing "people's medicine." Ehrenreich and English argue that people's medicine was "a more humane, empirical approach to healing" while the new male-dominated medical elite adhered to "untested doctrines and ritualistic practices" and "served the ruling class, both medically and politically" (ibid.:4–5). This character of biomedicine led Ehrenreich and English to conclude that "professionalism in medicine is nothing more than the institutionalization of a male upper-class monopoly" (ibid.:42). Furthermore, they argue that the male-dominated medical profession derives its power from "deep-rooted institutional sexism . . . sustained by a class system which supports male power." This view of medicine as based on patriarchy has led many radical feminists to adhere to a populist viewpoint and distrust all centralized solutions: Neither big government nor big business works for the interest of the individual consumer. For example, Ehrenreich and English see women's empowerment as residing in an unregulated market where women can together build up their strength in the form of a strong feminist consumer movement (ibid.:43).[3]

Yet, there is another essentialist approach to professions, an approach that has been prevalent in research and theories on women leadership and management and organizational theory. This view also stresses the dissimilarities between men and women but valorizes women's difference in experience, values, ways of behaving, feeling, and thinking. With reference to management and organizational theories, Alvesson and Billing (1997:161–70) distinguish between a moderate and a strong position on this issue, positions they call "the special contribution" and "alternative values" positions, respectively. The moderate position holds that women can contribute something special to organizations and that women possess qualifications complementary to men's. Women can bring qualities that men seem to lack. Such female qualities are an empathic, people-oriented, and democratic leadership style that can make organizations less hierarchical and make the workplace climate more democratic and team-work oriented (Reskin and Roos 1990:50–51). In the area of management, the argument has been that the old authoritarian and hierarchical management style is no longer functional and that organizational efficiency demands a new management style that conforms to female qualities—communication skills, teamwork-building, cooperation, and networking. The assumptions have been that if women are brought into management positions, they will bring these new values and behaviors to the management of the organization.

The strong position or the so-called alternative-values position emphasizes the radically conflicting differences between male and female values and behaviors. Within feminist theory, this perspective has been called cultural feminism (Evans 1995), which is defined as "the ideology of a female nature or female essence reappropriated by feminists themselves in an effort to validate undervalued female attributes" (Alcoff 1988:408). This reevaluation of women's traditional position has resulted in a view that defines women by their activities and attributes in the present culture. It claims that women have a different culture and rationality than men because of their early childhood experiences. The female culture is a special bond that women through their bodily experiences and caring as mothers have in common. This view attributes different psychological characteristics to women than to men (Evans 1995:77; James 1997; Lorber 1998:125). But it is also a view on work and organizations that can easily lead to a defense of separatism and segregation. The argument here is that women should not lose their own culture by integrating into the work culture of men but should adhere to their own values and interests and thereby achieve their own goals as women (see Alvesson and Billing 1997:168).

Some, however, have pointed out that these female-specific skills are not so much inherent in women as grounded on a material base: a patriarchal gender system assigning women a subordinated position in society (Billing 1997; Lorber 1998). A valorization of women's culture and specific skills associated with that culture only results in an acceptance and further confirmation of not only the traditional gender categories but also the very gender system the female culture is grounded on. Furthermore, Billing (1997), in her analysis of the view on women's specific skills in management, suggests that traditional female skills in the private sphere cannot automatically be assumed to be transferable or even to work in the world of management. It is more often the case that women's human-relations skills are recognized and constitute the reason for their promotion to those kind of managerial positions in which they have to solve the value and human-relations conflicts between employees and top management (Reskin and Roos 1990:51). Meanwhile male managers are left undisturbed, to concentrate on the crucial economic and technical aspects of the organization.

## CONCLUSIONS

This chapter has covered two issues related to the debates on gender and the medical profession.

The first section reviewed the underlying gendered aspects of major theoretical perspectives on the power of the medical profession. These perspectives and their underlying assumptions about gender are summarized in Figure 2.1. In the functionalist approach, women have been invisible members of the profession, since the focus in this genre of research has been on the gender-neutral professional norms and professional behavior of the physician. The physician is portrayed as guided by a science- and service-orientation, two underlying core values of the institutionalized role pattern of the physician (Parsons 1951). The professional traits, however, bear a close resemblance to male gender traits. Any female-gendered attributes have by definition not been part of the role of a professional, but have been seen as attitudes and attributes belonging to the private sphere of the family. Although the functionalist perspective has had a marginal status as a theoretical framework in research on professions during the past thirty years, it has still been very influential because of its socialization theory. This theory explains the adoption of roles and identities as a process of primary and secondary socialization. The focus is on inculcation of certain values and on the individual as the product of those normative guidelines—a viewpoint that early resulted in a criticism of the "oversocialized" notion of human behavior (Wrong 1961).

The interactionist approach, as represented in the work of Hughes (1958) and later of Goffman (1959, 1961), focuses on the social drama of work. A profession is associated with a certain master status and its auxiliary traits. Those who do not fit this master status have to negotiate with clients (and colleagues) to establish a relationship based on professional expertise and service. The master status of the medical profession seems still to be male gendered, which has posed problems for women entering into and practicing in it.

The neo-Marxian perspective has indirectly brought up gender as an issue by pointing out that women tend to have the lower-level, low-prestige, and low-income positions in the health care industry. According to Navarro (1976), women constitute the working class of health care, while women physicians are seen as class allies of medical men tied to the interests of the capitalist class. McKinlay has, however, refuted this class association of the physicians and instead predicted an increasing concentration of a capital-intensive health care industry—a corporate and bureaucratized medicine—and a simultaneous "proletarianization" of physicians. This "transformation of doctoring" and "loss of the golden age of doctoring," as this process has been characterized, denotes a change whereby doctors are becoming employees in large bureaucratic health care organizations. This view interprets health care as part of the economic system in society, which in the words of Berliner (1982) has proceeded from a cottage-industry production to a factory mode of production to its current stage of corporate medicine.

By many non-Marxists, the proletarianization of physicians has been called by another term denoting the same phenomenon: "feminization." This term has been used in a pejorative sense to indicate the transformation of a previously male-dominated profession, with the number of women increasing at the same time that the status of the profession is declining. Both scholars and the general debate have pondered over the causality: Do men leave a profession because it is becoming lower status as women enter? Or have women been able to enter because the profession is no longer considered a high-status profession? This question has been addressed in Reskin and Roos's (1990) study of long-term changes in the U.S. labor market. Their queueing theory views gender segregation as a consequence of two processes—labor queues and job queues, whereby employers rank workers and workers rank jobs—and both are shaped by gendered processes and practices.

The neo-Weberian perspective has been used by researchers to make visible the professionalization process and professional power that has granted a profession its monopoly. Some scholars have pointed to the gendered character of this process and the gendered character of the professional project of biomedicine. The professional-dominance view of professions originally proposed by Freidson (1970) resembles the neo-Weberian view, and a recent addition to this kind of perspective on professions has been Abbott's (1988) view about the jurisdictional power of professions.

The gendered character of medicine has been advanced by some of the social constructionists and postmodernists. In contrast to the emphasis on structural factors and the concerted group action toward a collective goal, represented by neo-Weberian scholars, the social constructionists and the postmodernists privilege gendered social practices—exemplified by the latter as the medical discourse—as the shapers of the power relations and character of health care. The early social constructionists presented medicine as a mechanism of social control (Zola 1972) and as an ever-expanding enterprise that subjugated a variety of social behaviors under its jurisdiction, a phenomenon called medicalization (Conrad 1992, 2000). Feminists drew attention to the gendered character of medicalization, because much of this labeling concerned women's bodies and reproduction. Feminist sociologists in this area have tended to focus on social practices and certain frameworks that—because of their gendered character—influence the diagnoses, treatment, and client-physician relationship of, particularly, women patients (Lorber 1997; Katz-Rothman 1998).

The postmodernists focus on representations and discourses that concern health and illness, but do not grant the biomedical discourse—i.e., the medical profession—ultimate power. The medical profession is not, as the neo-Weberians see it, a group that is above all propelled in its actions to guard its self-interest, but more, as the neo-Marxists see it, a servant of a broader disciplinary regime. Although the medical profession currently has a hegemonic position in most Western societies, this does not mean that it has authoritative power. Alternative medical and lay discourses challenge as well as endorse the biomedical discourse, and hence there is nothing intrinsically gendered in the biomedical discourse. As Lupton (1997) points out, the postmodern position, notably the Foucauldian, on the power of the profession views the power of health care not as monolithic but as fragmented. As Lupton (ibid.) notes, according to the Foucauldian framework, it is impossible to demedicalize the body and give the power back to the patients. As Lupton suggests, the demedicalized body is not a more authentic mode of subjectivity and embodiment but merely a different frame of reference. For Foucault then, the medical discourse and medical gaze exerted by medical practitioners is not as intentional as in the other theoretical frameworks presented above. Instead, it is connected to a broader regime of social control that is dispersed and works through institutions, various professions, agencies, and the self-regulatory practices of the individual himself or herself (Lupton 1997:100; Broom and Woodward 1996; Oinas 1998).

The second section of this chapter provided an overview of those sociological studies that have explicitly addressed the issue of women's position and career in professions and organizations. Here, the existence of normative and structural barriers has been viewed as the mechanism whereby women's underrepresentation in the profession as a whole or in certain ranks of medicine can be explained. This view follows the contingent approach to gender and medicine, according to which medicine is fundamentally gender neutral. For historic reasons there still remain barriers to or imbalances in women's representation. When the reasons for the imbalance have been identified and acted upon, the increasing number of women in the lower ranks of medicine will slowly but steadily move up to the higher ranks of medicine.

Those who espouse the embedded approach argue that women's status in professions or organizations is not merely a numerical question of their representation but of certain structures and cultural worlds characterized by masculine values and behaviors. According to this view, medicine is not a gender-neutral enterprise but characterized by gendered processes and social practices.

A third approach is the essentialist, which presents medicine as a universal patriarchal culture, and women as united by a common female culture. This cultural approach can provide a forceful reason for feminist advocacy but it can also result in a marginalization of women, and can restructure them into their own sphere.

The theories presented in this chapter provide various frameworks for analyzing and understanding the medical profession and women's position in it. The difficulty arises when these theories are applied to specific societies. Most of the theories have emerged in and hold for U.S. society, which has a medical profession and a health care system markedly different from the European ones. A comparative study of women physicians therefore confronts the alleged universality of the U.S. theories about the transformation of medicine and the medical profession. The subsequent chapters will describe and compare the entry and the careers of women physicians in three different settings: the U.S., the Scandinavian, and the Russian/Soviet health care systems. I will use the concepts and theoretical perspectives above as analytical tools in order to compare and highlight the specific features of the position that women physicians have achieved in the medical profession in the three societal settings. I will also look at what kind of feminist agendas have been associated with women physicians' tasks in health care.

## NOTES

1. For Parsons, the physician is a male, which at the time he was writing certainly reflected the demographic character of the U.S. medical profession. Parsons defines the physician's major task: "The role of the physician centers on *his* responsibility for the welfare of the patient in the sense of facilitating *his* recovery from illness to the best of the physician's ability" (1951:447, italics added). Here Parsons describes not only the physician but also the patient in male gender terms. The gendering of the professions is even more explicit in his essay on the professions and social structure, in which he distinguishes the "professional man" from the "business man" (Parsons 1949:186–88). Parsons portrays the underlying motives of their behaviors as different: the former is an altruistic servant of his clients, the latter pursues his own self-interest. Parsons argues, "*Professional men* have been thought of standing above these sordid [egoistic] considerations, devoting their lives to 'service' of *their fellow men*" (ibid.:194, italics added).

2. In his early work, Freidson, like Parsons, constantly uses the masculine gender in his discussions of the characteristics and behavior of both the physician and the patient. For example, in the description of solo practice as the typical mode of practice in the United States, Freidson concludes that "this involves a man working by *himself* in an office which *he* secures and equips with *his* own capital, with patients who have freely chosen *him* as their personal physician and for whom *he* assumes responsibility" (1970:91, italics added). Furthermore, in describing the lay referral network, colleague-dependent practice, the community and hospital physicians, Freidson consistently uses the masculine (e.g., ibid.:109–10, 307–9); and when women in the health labor force are referred to, they are treated as nurses and paramedical personnel. But in his later works, in the 1980s, Freidson uses the plural in referring to the profession's incumbents, thus avoiding gendering them. On such occasions that he does use the singular, the physician is referred to as "he or she" (e.g., Freidson 1985:28).

3. When Ehrenreich and English (and also others in the feminist health movement) were writing on medicine, there was an essentialist slant to their valorization of the woman patient's perspective (see Lorber 1997:80–81). The radical feminists later adopted a more nuanced view on women and medicine and today acknowledge diversity among women and men as patients and doctors.

# 3

# Women's Entry into Medicine and Medical Practice in the United States

## INTRODUCTION

The purpose of this chapter is to provide an overview of women's position in the medical profession in the United States. In the next two chapters women's medical careers in two other contexts—the Scandinavian countries and Russia/Soviet Union—will be presented. From a sociological point of view, the three social contexts will inform us about the collective mobility of women as they have aspired to a career in medicine. The argument advanced in this and the subsequent two chapters is that underlying the "heroine story" of the pioneering women in medicine were certain modes of production and concomitant structural constraints or opportunity structures, which not only influenced the careers of the individual pioneering women but also signaled the collective mobility of women in modern medicine as a social organization. In many countries, the admission of women to medical studies became a litmus test of the general societal view of women's capacities to pursue higher education. At issue was a traditional view of woman's biological destiny, which was assumed to set certain limits for her intellectual potential. Not only feminists but, more important, profeminist male mentors and administrative and political decision-makers challenged this notion and propagated a view of women that harbored the ideas of both the Enlightenment and contemporary liberalism and its views on individual rights. Still others argued that women's specific task in medicine was due to women's gender-typical skills, a view based on essentialist notions of femininity. The latter view was in many cases a common denominator among the conservatives and more progressive proponents, a notion that resulted in the admission of women into special tracks or programs designed for them. Nevertheless, despite the emergence of coeducational programs, women medical graduates entered a health care system that restricted women's practice to certain gender-specific specialties and practices.

In the nineteenth century, women's entry into medicine was predominantly a question of overcoming the formal barriers to women's admission to universities. The United States and Russia created temporary solutions by instituting gender-segregated medical education for women in the 1850s and 1870s, respectively. In international terms, the gender segregation of medical education opened early the practice of medicine to a sizeable group of women in the United States and Russia. By contrast, the coeducational policies adopted in the Scandinavian countries meant a later start for women as medical practitioners. Yet, the developments in the proportion and representation of women in the ranks of medicine in the twentieth century cannot be explained merely by these different early educational policies. Later, certain patterns of segregation and hierarchization of medical work by gender not only remained but became increasingly visible as new areas of medicine developed.

During the twentieth century, medicine as a mode of production followed the economic development of the rest of the society. According to a neo-Marxist perspective (Navarro 1976; Berliner 1982), medicine can be divided into three modes of production: cottage industry, factory mode, and corporate. In the first phase, *cottage industry production*, fee-for-service and the physician as private entrepreneur were predominant. The second phase, which followed the *factory mode of production* in the rest of society, was the rise of hospital medicine. In the social organization of medicine, a growing internal differentiation and hierarchical structure emerged. Some recent researchers in the health field have characterized this factory mode as a Fordist regime—a system of mass production of standardized products and an expanding market (Nettleton 1995:216). The characteristics of this large-scale, capital-intensive production perhaps better match the third phase in health care, which U.S. researchers have called *corporate medicine*. Corporate medicine has been seen as dominated by powerful economic forces resulting in a concentration of ownership in health care and loss of control over work by physicians (see also Starr 1982; Coburn 1999). Yet, most European countries have witnessed a decentralization rather than a centralization of the structure of health care and the welfare state since the mid-1980s. In these countries, the term post-Fordism has been seen as a more accurate description of the health care market. In a post-Fordist regime, the production becomes decentralized to respond to new and different consumer choices and demands. As a consequence, the health care labor force has to adapt to these changing markets, which are more consumer driven than profession driven (Nettleton 1995:217; Twaddle 1999:52).

The argument presented in this chapter and the next two chapters is that women's position in medicine has at all times captured the structural change in medicine. The study of women physicians illuminates the major transformations of medicine as a social organization and as a profession. These transformations have had gendered implications. During the various phases in the mode of production of medicine, men physicians have been in the forefront of the new structure of medicine, while women physicians, as a less powerful group in the profession, have practiced in the less prestigious or more routinized parts of medical work. Here the concept of queueing—both of labor markets and jobs by gender—denotes the gendered processes that give rise to the gender-segregated hierarchies of work (Reskin and Roos 1990; Acker 1992). This chapter highlights the importance of certain external and structural conditions that have shaped women physicians' opportunities to advance or constraints on advancing in their profession [external meaning economic conditions, structural meaning conditions shaping job opportunities in the healthcare field]. In some countries, the structural conditions have meant new career opportunities, while in others they have implied subtle new structural obstacles to advancing in the profession.

This chapter will provide a descriptive, historical account of the educational opportunities available for women to study medicine in the nineteenth century in the United States and the social and political conditions that influenced the early and later careers for women in medicine in the twentieth century.

## THE FIRST GENERATION OF AMERICAN WOMEN PHYSICIANS

In the United States professions are more or less laborious, more or less profitable; but they are never either high or low: every honest calling is honorable.

—Alexis de Tocqueville, *Democracy in America*

The first woman to practice medicine in the United States, but trained by apprenticeship, was Harriot Hunt in 1835. More than a decade later, Elizabeth Blackwell graduated from Geneva Medical College, New York, in 1849 (Walsh 1977). She was followed by six women, who graduated from Western Reserve College in Cleveland between 1852 and 1856, and Mary Harris Thompson, who got her medical degree from the Chicago Medical College in 1870. The first African-American woman, Rebecca Lee, received her degree from New England Female Medical College in 1864 (More 1999:4). In 1860, 200 or 300 women were practicing medicine—about 0.4 percent of the physicians in the United States. In 1870, there were 600 or 700. After that the numbers began to rise fast: in 1890, there were 4,557 women physicians

(4.4 percent), of whom 115 were black (ibid.:5). In 1900 there were 7,387 women physicians (5.6 percent), and by 1910 they were 9,015 (6 percent), figures that are comparatively high for that time (Walsh 1977:186).

Three indigenous conditions seem to have made for the much earlier presence of women physicians in U.S. society than in most European countries, where physicians enjoyed a licensed and state-regulated professional position. Mid-nineteenth-century U.S. medicine was characterized by (1) the lack of licensing requirements in most states, (2) the pluralistic or "sectarian" character of medicine, and (3) the existence of separate women's medical colleges.

First, the political and social climate of the Jacksonian era was characterized by antielitist sentiments and populism. This was an agrarian-based protest movement in the 1840s, which objected to tendencies to the emergence of centralized power and elitist authority in America (Hofstadter 1955). In medicine, this sentiment was expressed as a hostility to licensing, which was seen as a measure to create a privileged elite of regular physicians. By 1850, many states had revoked licensing requirements as a prerequisite for medical practice. This created an age of pluralistic medicine, with medical schools providing a large variety of therapy traditions (Stevens 1976:26–30; Rothstein 1972; Starr 1982).[1]

Second, the disillusionment with regular physicians and the heroic medicine that they practiced brought about a rise in the market of alternative therapies. Such therapies were often less harmful and more oriented toward prevention (Rothstein 1972). Among them were those that promoted herbal remedies (e.g., the Thomsonians, the eclectics) and homeopathy. The sectarian medical colleges provided a rather short education, on the average eight or nine months long, in contrast to the five years of study required in most medical schools in Europe at the time (ibid.; Bonner 1988:62). The sectarian medical colleges welcomed women, whereas most medical schools of regular medicine remained closed to women until the turn of the century. Some of those sectarian schools that graduated women before 1850 were Central (eclectic), Syracuse (eclectic), Western Homeopathic, and Western Reserve (homeopathic) (Rogers 1990:293; Morantz-Sanchez 1985:49).

The following figures illuminate how far the regular medical schools restricted the admission of women. Among the 600 or 700 women physicians practicing in 1870, only eight had graduated from coeducational, regular medical colleges. By 1893, only 37 out of 105 regular medical schools accepted women (ibid.:65). For example, the University of California began to admit women in 1869, the University of Michigan opened its doors to women medical students in 1871, and Syracuse University in 1870. Furthermore, the Medical Department at Johns Hopkins University received a large donation attached to which was the condition that women be admitted on equal terms with men (Moldow 1987:7–8) and women began promptly to be admitted in 1893. The Cornell University Medical School followed in 1899, while the medical schools at Harvard, Pennsylvania, Yale, and Columbia remained closed to women until early 1900 (Bonner 1988:71). One of the last holdouts against coeducation was the College of Physicians of Philadelphia, founded in 1787. It eventually became coeducational in 1932—after a history of 145 years as an all-male organization (Marks and Beatty 1972:114). (See Table 3.1.)

Third, separate women's medical colleges and hospitals were a feature of the education of women physicians in the United States in the nineteenth century. For example, the first women's medical college—the Woman's Medical College of Pennsylvania—was established by the Quakers in 1850; the New England Female Medical College of the New York Infirmary was originally founded in 1850 to train midwives but became a regular medical college for women in 1868; and Women's Medical College of Baltimore was founded in 1882 (Walsh 1977; Drachman 1984, 1986; Moldow 1987:6; Bonner 1988; Morantz-Sanchez 1985). These institutions were part of regular medicine but were based on separatism as an operating principle in U.S. society, where the public sphere was controlled by men.

As Drachman (1984:200) shows, one of the early women physicians, the Polish-born but U.S.-educated Marie Zakrzewska adopted the strategy of separatism for women's clinical training and practice out of necessity as women were barred from hospital practice in mainstream male medicine. Yet, Zakrzewska's conviction was that by establishing an institution—the all-woman-staffed New England Hospital for Women and Children founded in 1862—parallel to the one in the male world, women would learn the skills of male medicine and be invited to enter it. In Zakrzewska's worldview, the surest path to integration was through the strategy of separation. Hence, her medical institution was not founded in opposition to male medicine but as an accommodation to the separatism prevailing in society at large. While her hospital worked apart from mainstream male medicine, she wanted it to become an acknowledged part of the mainstream. But as Drachman (ibid.) shows, the rising expectations of a younger generation of women physicians resulted in a challenge of the separatism strategy since they felt constrained by the limited possibilities of their education and practice. Their separate sphere was not only perceived as secondary to the men's, but they were also cut off from resources to develop female-based institutions.

The coeducational opportunities for medical studies available in Europe gave the more career-oriented American women a chance to achieve educational equity with men. The medical school of the University of Zurich had opened its doors to women in 1864, and the medical school of the University of Paris in 1868. The opening of university education to

Table 3.1.   Women's Entry into Medicine: Comparing the United States, the Scandinavian Countries, and Russia/Soviet Union

| Country | Access to medical education | First woman physician | Percentage of women physicians | | |
| --- | --- | --- | --- | --- | --- |
| | | | 1910 | 1950 | 1990 |
| U.S. | Apprenticeship Geneva Medical College Era of pluralistic medicine, 1850–1910 | Harriot Hunt, 1835 Elizabeth Blackwell, 1849 Few coeducational medical schools, but sectarian and women's medical schools women; European-trained women physicians | 6 | 6 | 17 |
| Scandinavia | Coeducational medical studies | | | | |
| Sweden | 1870 | Karolina Widerström, 1888 | | 9 | 34 |
| Finland | 1871 | Rosina Heikel, 1878 | 3 | 21 | 42 |
| Denmark | 1875 | Nielsene Nielsen, 1885 | | 10 | 26 |
| Norway | 1882 | Marie Spångberg, 1893 | | 10 | 23 |
| Russia | Women audit medical courses in St. Petersburg, 1859–1864 Women study medicine at University of Zurich and University of Paris, 1864–1872 Women's medical courses in St. Petersburg, 1872–1887 Women's Medical Institute, 1895–1917 | Nadezda Suslova, 1867 691 women graduated 2,804 women graduated | 10 | 77 | 69 |

women in France and Switzerland started a wave of migration of women. Russian and American women were among the first to graduate from the medical schools in France and Switzerland (Bonner 1988, 1989). Medicine was one of the major subjects that drew women to the University of Zurich. By 1914, around seven thousand foreign women had studied medicine there (Bonner 1988:62). Susan Dimock was the first American woman to earn a medical degree abroad in 1871, and the fourth foreign woman to do so at Zurich. Other women followed. From 1870 to 1914, fifty-seven

American women pursued their medical studies there. In 1871, another American woman, Mary Corinna Putnam, earned her medical degree at the University of Paris. She had been the first foreign woman admitted to its faculty of medicine, and the second woman to be graduated from there with a medical degree (Bonner 1988:58–59, 1989).

American women were not alone in this sojourn—men went as well, but for different reasons. Women went to get a basic medical education because in the United States few of them had access to clinical study and to patients. By contrast, most men went to improve their knowledge in a clinical specialty and fundamental laboratory science (Bonner 1988:65). Furthermore, for the men Germany was the major destination; but women were not able to study medicine there until 1908 (in Prussia). One woman, Dorothea Christiane Erxleben-Leporin, had received her medical degree in 1754 from the University of Halle; but the university's pietist mission made this first case an exception to the rule (Geyer-Kordesh 1983:25).

As regular U.S. medical schools gradually began to allow women to study medicine, women's medical colleges and hospitals began, in the late 1890s and early 1900s, to close their doors. This was an era of trust in science and a refurbishing of the higher educational system in the United States. In U.S. medicine, the Flexner report of 1910 consolidated the biomedical and allopathic paradigm of medicine and education according to a European and notably German model. The Flexner report also pruned the sectarian, women's, and black medical colleges from the list of institutions to be accredited as high-quality medical schools (Berliner 1975; Rothstein 1972; Stevens 1976; Starr 1982). While the country had 162 medical schools in existence in 1906, only ninety-five were operating a decade later (*JAMA* 1923:553).

As Walsh (1990) notes, the assumption has been that the all-women medical schools were closed on account of the Flexner report. Flexner (1910:178) himself shows, however, that only three of the seventeen medical colleges for women remained in 1909, when he did his evaluation of the quality of the education offered by the medical schools in the United States and Canada.

In his report of 1910, Flexner devoted a whole chapter, "The Medical Education of Women," to pondering the status of women in U.S. medical education. Contrary to the negative slant attributed to his views on women's medical colleges in later literature, Flexner comments in positive terms on woman's role in medicine:

> Woman has so apparent a function in certain medical specialties and seemingly so assured a place in general medicine under some obvious limitations that the struggle for wider educational opportunities for the sex was predestined to an early success in medicine. (ibid.)

But Flexner is perplexed by the declining number of women studying medicine: 946 women studied at coeducational schools in 1904, as opposed to 752 in 1909; and the figures for women's medical schools show the same trend: 183 students in 1904, and 169 students in 1909. Flexner seems well aware of the potential barriers for women as their own schools and hospitals developed into integrated institutions. He emphasizes the need for women to be granted internships on equal terms with men:

> In the general need of more liberal support for medical schools, it would appear that large sums, as far as specially available for the medical education of women, would accomplish most if used to develop coeducational institutions, in which their benefits would be shared by men, without loss to women students; but it must be added, if separate medical schools and hospitals are not to be developed for women, *interne privileges must be granted to women on the same terms as to men.* (ibid.:179, emphasis added)

A number of alternative interpretations have been presented for the sudden dominance of allopathic medicine. Some historians (Rothstein 1972) interpret this radical decrease in the number of medical schools as a product of the growth of scientific knowledge and the emergence of scientifically valid medical therapies, a development that made the sectarians less attractive to a clientele demanding a scientific approach. Others (Berliner 1975, 1986) interpret the professional dominance of scientific or biomedicine as a result of the backing of powerful industrialists and professional circles in America.

According to the feminist interpretation, scientific medicine affirmed a male-dominated, biomedical view of illness, which defined women's traditional skills and medical knowledge as unscientific. Scientific medicine thus became a male-dominated enterprise (Ehrenreich and English 1973). The later integration of women into regular medical education and the ranks of allopathic medicine has been interpreted by Drachman (1986) and Walsh (1977) as a co-option of women into a male-dominated structure of medicine. Women physicians lost their constituency—women and children—and control over their own health care institutions, but were still assigned the same work. As Drachman (1986:59) argues, separatism persisted, though in new forms—within the newly integrated profession and under the premise of mainstream male-dominated medicine.

Other feminist scholars have tried to go beyond this oppression/victimization argument and privileged the various strategies that women physicians as active agents used to attain their own goals in spite of their marginalized position (e.g., Morantz-Sanchez 1985, 1990; Freedman 1979; More 1999).The complexity of the issue has been portrayed in the case studies by Drachman (1984), Morantz-Sanchez (1985), and More (1999), who have tried to reinstate women physicians as agents in rather than as victims of a male-dominated medical profession and organization of medicine. They have argued that the first generation of women physicians had a feminist collective consciousness and worked for women's health issues, along with public health and social reform, to advance the position of poor women and children. Constrained by the male values of professionalism and the ideology of domesticity and separatism, women physicians became involved in public health and social reform and used their scientific expertise to improve the health and well-being of women and children. This collective feminist or female consciousness was a feature of the pioneering women physicians, a shared consciousness that came to be expressed as a maternalist discourse. This discourse, which Morantz-Sanchez (1985) has called "scientific motherhood" and More (1999) "moral motherhood," channeled women into gender-specific health care settings. Women physicians began to work for dispensaries and special hospitals for women and children. As these endeavors in the private and voluntary sector of health care became more and more marginalized, women physicians began to work within the public health efforts that were the remnants of the social reforms of the progressive era. The last effort to save this social reform ethos was the Sheppard-Towner Act of 1921, which will be examined in the next section. As women physicians were advancing a public health agenda—to improve the health of working women and the health of children—they found themselves marginalized in the professionalized medicine created by the Flexner report. U.S. medicine was moving slowly but steadily toward a science- and university-based education and one where clinical training became a crucial part of the education of physicians. The professionally oriented women physicians joined forces, and in 1915 the Medical Women's National Association (in 1937 to be renamed the American Medical Women's Association) was founded (More 1999:124).

## WOMEN PHYSICIANS IN THE UNITED STATES IN THE TWENTIETH CENTURY

There were certainly many societal factors outside medicine that influenced women's position in general in the family and the economy and therefore indirectly came to influence women's search for higher education in general and for a career in medicine in particular. The analysis in this chapter is, however, limited to the factors intrinsic to the U.S. health care system and medicine. This narrow approach is deliberately chosen in order to highlight certain structures that might have advanced or hindered women's numbers and careers in U.S. medicine.

Table 3.2.    Women Physicians in the United
States, 1860–2010

| Year | Number | Percentage of total physicians |
|------|--------|-------------------------------|
| 1860 | 200 | 0.4 |
| 1890 | 4,557 | 4.4 |
| 1900 | 7,387 | 5.6 |
| 1910 | 9,015 | 6.0 |
| 1920 | 7,219 | 5.0 |
| 1930 | 6,825 | 4.4 |
| 1940 | 7,708 | 4.6 |
| 1950 | 11,823 | 6.1 |
| 1960 | 15,672 | 6.0 |
| 1970 | 25,507 | 7.7 |
| 1980 | 54,284 | 11.6 |
| 1990 | 104,194 | 16.9 |
| 1999 | 182,122 | 23.4 |
| 2000 | — | 24.1 |
| 2010 | — | 29.4 |

Source:   Walsh (1977:186), Roback et al. (1986:19,
25), Kletke et al. (1990:301), Pasko and Seidman (1999:23), www.ama-assn.org (2000).

Coeducation in regular medical schools gave women a chance in principle to enter medicine on equal terms with men. In the beginning, informal quotas and restrictions in the admission of women seem still to have
been maintained (Walsh 1977:243, 1990). As Table 3.2 shows, the proportion of women physicians remained largely unchanged between 1900 and
1960: Women constituted 6 percent of the U.S. physicians. In fact, the percentage declined in the 1930s and 1940s, when, too, the number of physicians declined from the number active in the profession in 1910.

The following two sections will address two issues. The first section
examines how the rise of hospital medicine influenced women physicians'
position in the profession, and the second section describes the practice
profile of women physicians during the era of corporate medicine, particularly in the late 1990s.

## Women Physicians in the Age of Hospital Medicine

Most of nineteenth-century U.S. medicine had a cottage industry character. It was pursued by independent practitioners in an entrepreneurial
fashion, and medical technology was restricted to what was included in
the doctor's black bag. It was during this cottage industry era that women

entered medicine, but medical practice was institutionalized into a male and a female pathway. Women physicians took care of women and children predominantly, and the success of their services lay chiefly in the practice of preventive medicine. Their practice, especially that of women who treated the lower classes, did not challenge men physicians. This type of practice was legitimated by the general ideology of "scientific" or "moral" motherhood prevalent in America at the end of the nineteenth and beginning of the twentieth century (Morantz-Sanchez 1985:22; More 1999:70).

The kind of holistic and preventive perspective that women had harbored was increasingly recognized as the public health perspective during the 1910s. The Flexner report set U.S. medicine on a new path: toward a science- and university-based education with concomitant clinical training. The professionalization of U.S. medicine had begun. But U.S. medical education had witnessed a surge of entrants to its existing medical colleges: In 1900, 25,171 students attended U.S. medical colleges, and in 1904 the number was 28,142 (*JAMA* 1923:549). Although the effects of the Flexner report became evident in the enrollment at medical schools—there were only about 13,000 students enrolled at the end of 1910s—the medical market was still characterized by competition for patients in the 1920s due to the "overproduction" of physicians during the previous decade.

It is against the backdrop of this "oversupply" of medical practitioners that the resistance toward a public health agenda in general and toward the Sheppard-Towner Act in particular has to be seen (see also More 1999; Brandt and Gardner 2000). The passage of the Sheppard-Towner Act in 1921—a year after American women had gained the right to vote—seemed a victory for a feminist agenda in medicine: The act provided matching federal funds to state health departments' initiatives in the area of infant and maternity health during a period of five years. By 1927, forty-three states had established child health bureaus (More 1999:153). The act was renewed in 1927 for two years, but no renewal was granted by the Congress in 1929 (Rothman 1978; Skocpol 1992). Nevertheless, this act was important since it was the predecessor to Title V of the Social Security Act of 1935, which provided the platform for later national programs in maternal and child health.

As several observers have suggested (Rothman 1978; More 1999; Brandt and Gardner 2000) organized medicine showed little interest in supporting the public health endeavors in maternal and child health. A glance at the editorials and articles on the theme of prevention and public health in the *Journal of the American Medical Association* in the 1920s gives a clear indication of what was at issue. The public health clinics constituted a threat to the private general practitioner, who was challenged both by the rural and city public health centers and by the emerging hospital medicine. In the journal of organized medicine, women physicians' work in the domain of public health was invisible. Instead, the leading articles on this issue pondered how the medical profession could gain control over the preventive and public health initiatives. Obviously the emergence of public health departments and their public health administrators was perceived as a threat to the market and the autonomy of the profession. A number of articles (e.g., Dickie 1923; Dodson 1923) suggested the need for integrating preventive medicine into the medical curriculum so that future private practitioners would provide the kind of services to their individual patients that now were offered as a public health service. The political undertone was evident—mostly tacit but sometimes also quite explicit. For example, one leading article on the relationship between the medical profession and health authorities suggested:

> Rather than the health department giving orders to the medical profession, it would be more seemly for the physician to give instructions to the health department. . . . The medical profession has too long permitted the laws dealing with health to be interpreted entirely by a public health executive. This should be changed and we, the physicians of the country, must see that it is done. (McLean 1921:827)

Another article written by the president of the Hospital Service Association of New York promoted the needs of social medicine but saw the physician as the expert on this perspective:

> The physician can and should become the law giver in social as well as individual ills. He, more than any one else, has opportunity to see life as it really is, stripped of illusions, and on the bedrock of truth. Certainly he is a surer guide in social affairs than some reformers with crude but well meaning specifics, or hysterical world-betterers who are liable to do more harm than good, in spite of benevolent intentions. (Chapin 1921:281)

In a leading article the president of the AMA (Billings 1923:524) gave a similar message when he pondered the importance of the general practitioner in the larger social transformation of U.S. society and medicine:

> The American family home has been and must continue to be the very foundation of this nation. Bolshevistic socialism, anarchy and public discord cannot exist in a nation of family homes. The integrity and perpetuation of this nation is dependent chiefly on the maintenance of family life; and the continuance of the family home demands the preservation of the family physician, the general practitioner.

The AMA did not endorse the Sheppard-Towner Act in 1929. The act was considered a failure since there had been no major changes in infant and maternal mortality rates while it was in force. An editorial on the issue in *JAMA* denounced the "resurrection of Sheppard-Townerism" and declared: "If the act stimulated the states in this manner [to provide welfare and hygiene services to mothers and infants] it accomplished its purpose and there is no reason for resurrecting it. If it did not, the act was a failure, and there is even less reason for doing so" (*JAMA* 1930:1240). But as More (1999:162) shows also, the Medical Women's National Association conformed to the new political climate and took a nonsupportive stance toward the renewal of the act as well as later proposals for a national health insurance.

By the mid-1920s the division of public health and biomedicine was a fact. This development was propelled by the professionalization of both medicine and public health. The two perspectives became institutionalized in separate schools: medicine and public health. The perspective of social medicine and public health became the scientific core knowledge of the nation's new schools of public health (Brandt and Gardner 2000:710). As More (1999:82) has noted, social reform at the turn of the century gave women physicians a career opportunity in public health, but by the 1930s the professionalization of public health also ended the era of women's stronghold in this area.

During the nineteenth century, hospital medicine was in the hands of voluntary organizations and had the character of charity medicine more than its later locus as an institution of medical science. In 1870s, there were only 170 hospitals in the United States, a figure that had increased to about 1,500 in 1904, and in 1925 to about 7,000 in cities alone (ibid.:105–6). As hospital medicine and the phase of the industrialization of medicine gained momentum after World War I, women physicians were left at the fringes of this development. While they had managed to get access to medical education and to work as solo-practitioners in cottage industry medicine, entry into hospital medicine required an internship and later affiliation with a hospital in order to treat its patients. As shown in the previous section of this chapter, Abraham Flexner (1910:178–79) was well aware of this barrier for women and recommended that they be granted internships on equal terms with men.

That internships and residencies became a new barrier for women's advancement in the medical profession has been amply documented. More (1999:109) shows that of the hospitals with AMA-approved internships in 1925, only 24 percent would consider women. This condition severely restricted women's career opportunities in medicine, especially since this was the time when hospital medicine in the United States took off. Drachman (1984) and More (1999:58) show in their case studies that early women physicians were excluded from this sphere, and the establishment of dispensaries for women and children in New York, Boston, Philadelphia, Baltimore, Rochester, and Washington, D.C., was a female strategy to overcome women's exclusion from the resources of male medicine. Yet, as hospital medicine became more resource intensive and a dominant practice pattern in U.S. medicine, the younger generation of women physicians realized that they could no longer stay outside this structure. In her case study of the New England Hospital for Women and Children, Drachman (1984) illustrates the conflict between the pioneering generation of women physicians and the younger generation. For the older generation, the gender-segregated pattern of hospital practice that had been established out of necessity was seen as a litmus test of the loyalty to a shared female culture as the younger generation became attracted to the professional standards and resources of male-dominated mainstream medicine (see also More 1999).

Thus, it was not the closure of women's medical schools and exclusion from coeducational schools that explains the later drop in the number of women physicians in the United States (see Table 3.2). Rather it was the professionalization of public health and of biomedicine and, especially, the rise of a new hierarchical and medical organization—the hospital—that became the barrier. In such a hierarchical system, as Lorber notes, it meant restriction of the opportunity for women physicians "to compete with the men for the scarce resources of the professional patronage system. . . . At the same time, they lost whatever advantage their sex had given them in the competition for patients" (1985:84).

For American women physicians, for various reasons the entry to hospital medicine was different from what it was for European women. The development of the modern hospital proceeded at a different pace and in a different path in U.S. society. In most of Europe, hospital physicians were employees. Private practitioners referred their patients to the hospital, where the hospital physicians took over the treatment. Furthermore, notably in Germany and France, the larger urban hospitals were connected to medical schools and their training of students and thus were, in the nineteenth century, the site of scientific medicine. By contrast, U.S. hospitals between 1870 and 1910 were mainly charity institutions (Starr 1982). After the Flexner report in 1910, efforts to increase the quality of U.S. medicine—both medical education and hospitals—put pressure on communities to redefine and reconstruct the task of the hospitals and to cater to a paying clientele. The U.S. hospitals, however, remained private or what has been called voluntary—that is, most of them worked on a nonprofit basis and were financed by local donations rather than by taxes, as in Europe. Stevens (1982) has pointed out that, before the depression, the U.S. nonprofit hospital system was not perceived as belonging to the "private market." The hospitals presented themselves as "public" institutions, since they were considered public utilities open to all and were run not for profit but as tax-exempt charity organizations.

In the United States, hospital physicians remained private practitioners rather than hospital employees. When a patient was hospitalized, those physicians who were affiliated with a local hospital could continue to serve their private patients in the hospital.

Over the past hundred years, the U.S. hospital system has undergone a profound change, more so than European hospitals. The U.S. hospital system has—because of its funding system and the autonomous status of the medical profession—been related to various external structures of power. The character and the layers of the power structures impinging on the organization of U.S. hospitals have been unraveled in one of the classics of medical sociology: Perrow's (1963) analysis of the goals and power structure of a hospital in an urban area and its transformation from 1885 to the early 1960s. This case study of one hospital can here serve as a heuristic device to illuminate the changes in the power structure of most U.S. hospitals. For our purposes it can also provide an insight into the conditions of hospital appointments for women physicians.

The kind of power exerted over the organization of the hospital can be divided into five phases, adapted here from Perrow's (1963) local study to the national level. The first period between 1885 and 1929 was a phase of *trustee dominance,* when the local charity leaders on the hospital board and its president ran the hospital. The second period, between 1929 and 1947, was a period of *medical dominance,* when the post-Flexner effects of improving the quality of hospital services legitimated the physicians' authority and control of the hospital. The third period, between 1947 and 1965, was a time of *administrative challenge,* when third-party payers enter the scene and the hospital came to need a hospital administrator to handle the different power and authority structures (doctors, trustees, third-party payers like Hill-Burton grants, instituted in 1946, and insurance companies like Blue Cross and Blue Shield, established in 1948). In 1965 began a fourth period of *multiple control,* when a number of federal programs—for example, Medicaid, Medicare, and the Community Health Planning Act—began to demand consumer participation in health planning and policymaking. The fifth period can be said to have emerged with the *rise of corporate medicine* in the mid-1970s (Starr 1982:429–30), which has consolidated the hospital system into large multihospital systems, increasingly profit-oriented and run by a corporate management. Since the mid-1980s, this development has accelerated and the practice of medicine in America has undergone a marked change.

During the phase of trustee dominance of hospitals (1885–1929), women of local prominence could by themselves or through their husbands influence the founding of hospitals. During the later phases, the hospital structure has been part of a male-dominated power structure. Research on the interlinks between the community power structure and the composition of hospital boards provides a further account of the over-lap between the economic structure and the hospital power structure in the United States in the 1960s and early 1970s (see, e.g., Elling 1963; Pfeffer 1973; Holloway, Artis, and Freeman 1963).

The rise of corporate medicine has been a challenge to the previous autonomous status of the medical profession in the delivery of its services. As for the medical profession, the implications of this latest "social transformation of American medicine" (Starr 1982) have been more closely reviewed in the literature on the sociology of professions and subsumed under the heading "proletarianization" (McKinlay and Arches 1985), "corporatization" (McKinlay and Stoeckle 1988), or "restratification" (Freidson 1985) of the U.S. medical profession. These perspectives were presented in the theoretical overview in Chapter 2.

## Medical Work and American Women Physicians in the Age of Corporate Medicine

During the first decade of the twentieth century, women constituted 6 percent of the physicians, only to decline in absolute and relative numbers over the next three decades. A rapid growth of the numbers of women physicians can be discerned since 1970, a development that has been further spurred by affirmative-action policies. The passage of Title IX of the Higher Education Act in 1972 banned discrimination in admission and salaries in any school receiving federal funds. This act and subsequent affirmative action programs improved the opportunities for women and members of minority groups to enter into and to advance in their career in medicine. The proportion of women entering medical school has increased rapidly since 1970. In 1999–2000, women constituted 46 percent of the cohort entering medical schools, compared to 28 percent in 1980, and 9 percent in 1970 (Relman 1989:1540; Chavkin 1997:733; Bickel 2000:10; Barzansky, Jonas, and Etzel 2000:1116). Already in the 1980s, Relman (1989) noted the changing demography of the medical profession, as he called attention to the decline in total applications by men—which fell by 50 percent from 1974 to 1989.

A closer look at the first-year medical students in U.S. allopathic medical schools reveals that among the first-year medical students in 1999–2000, 65 percent were white, 19 percent were Asian, 8 percent African-American, 7 percent Hispanic, and 1 percent Native-American. Women's representation varied considerably between these groups. The highest proportion of women first-year medical students was among African-Americans (66 percent), followed by Hispanics (47 percent), and by Native-Americans and Asians (46 percent). The lowest proportion of women was among whites (43 percent) (Barzansky et al. 2000:1117).

Table 3.3.   Distribution (%) of Physician Population by Type of Practice and Percentage of
Women, in the U.S. in 1996

| Practice type | All physicians | Percentage female |
|---|---|---|
| Employee | 42 | 23 |
| Solo | 28 | 11 |
| Self-employed group | 30 | 10 |
| Total | 100 | — |

Source:   Moser (1998:31).

In the U.S. health care system women physicians tend to work in different practice settings and specialties than men. Today the private and solo practice is no longer the predominant mode—a large proportion of U.S. physicians are employed in large practices (see Table 3.3). Women are self-employed less often than men in 1996: 11 percent of the solo and 10 percent of the self-employed physicians in group practice were women. The figures become more dramatic if women are looked at as a group, especially with the rise of corporate medicine in the 1980s. For example, 24 percent of U.S. physicians practiced as salaried employees in 1983, and the proportion had risen to 42 in 1996 and to 43 in 1997 (Kletke, Emmons, and Gillis 1996:557; Moser 1998:31).

This trend toward employee status was particularly evident among women physicians: In 1983, 44 percent of the women physicians were salaried and the percentage rose to 56 in 1997. The figures for male physicians were 22 percent in 1983 and 35 percent in 1997 [Kletke et al. 1996:558; American Medical Women's Association (AMWA) 2000:4].

Within and between specialties, women physicians are also differently distributed than men. Internal medicine, followed by family practice and general surgery, had the most men. The largest number of women was also in internal medicine (Table 3.4), followed by pediatrics and family practice. General surgery ranked tenth in number of women. This low ranking is also reflected in the percentage of women among practicing surgeons, as documented in Table 3.4.

In 1997, the highest proportions of women were found in pediatrics (46 percent), child psychiatry (39 percent), obstetrics and gynecology (32 percent), psychiatry and pathology (28 percent) (Table 3.4). The lowest proportion was found in general surgery (9 percent). Yet, women are making inroads in surgery. For example, in 1997, of the women surgeons, 49 percent were under thirty-five years old, as compared to 21 percent of the male surgeons (Pasko and Seidman 1999:45).

*Table 3.4.* Proportion (%) of Women in Selected
Specialties in the U.S. in 1997

| Type of specialty | Total physicians | Percentage female |
|---|---|---|
| Anesthesiology | 33,730 | 20 |
| Child psychiatry | 5,620 | 39 |
| Dermatology | 9,062 | 30 |
| Family practice | 64,611 | 25 |
| General practice | 16,835 | 15 |
| Internal medicine | 128,435 | 25 |
| Neurology | 11,714 | 19 |
| Obstetrics/gynecology | 39,257 | 32 |
| Ophthalmology | 17,822 | 13 |
| Pathology | 18,236 | 28 |
| Pediatrics | 55,427 | 46 |
| Psychiatry | 39,064 | 28 |
| Radiology | 8,142 | 12 |
| Surgery (general) | 40,935 | 9 |

*Source:* Pasko and Seidman (1999:20, 28).

The differences in practice settings and type of specialties tend to create economic inequalities between male and female physicians. In 1996, the median net income of physicians in the United States was $166,000 (Moser 1998:30), but men physicians earned considerably more than women: In 1996, the median net income of the men was $177,000; of the women, $120.000. This means that women's earnings were 68 percent of men's, a figure up slightly from 62 percent in 1986 (ibid.:35).

Although the income gap between men and women physicians has narrowed slightly over the past decade, few women were found in the highest income group in the profession. If the highest and lowest groups are defined as those in the highest and lowest net-income quartile (i.e., 25 percent), only 4 percent of those in the highest group were women, while 32 percent among those in the lowest were women (ibid.:34). A number of the characteristics of women's practice profile were obviously also common to the low-income physicians: For example, 58 percent were employees and 55 percent worked in a primary-care specialty. In contrast, a majority (53 percent) of those in the highest net-income quartiles worked in self-employed group practices. These figures are further illuminated by a nationwide survey of young U.S. physicians (forty-five years old, with two to nine years of practice experience) in 1990, a survey documenting the same income gap. The results showed that the gender gap in earnings was further explained by the time spent at work: Men reported working an average 62 hours per week for 47 weeks while women reported 51 hours per week for 46 weeks (Baker 1996:962).

In the 1990s, women physicians are not as well represented in nonpatient as in patient care. Table 3.5 shows the proportion of women among all physicians working in medical teaching, administration, and research in 1970, 1980, and 1997. Progress is slow. Women constitute a mere fifth of those working in these categories, but the figures have doubled between 1970 and 1997.

Two decades ago, in 1977–1978, 10 percent of medical faculty were women, and the proportions declined the higher up in the ranks one looked: 8 percent of assistant professors, 5 percent of associate professors, and 3 percent of full professors were women (Tesch, Wood, Helwig, and Nattinger 1995). As a curiosity it might be mentioned that, during this time, the Medical College of Pennsylvania, formerly Woman's Medical College, still had by far the largest percentage of women in each faculty category (Farrell, Witte, Holguin, and Lopez 1979:2809). In the 1990s, women have advanced slowly but progressively at the academic level of medicine. Although the process is slow, the American figures look more promising by far than those of the Scandinavian countries, to be shown in the next chapter. In 1999, women were 27 percent of full-time medical school faculty (Bickel 2000:10). The highest proportion was recorded in pediatrics (41%), and orthopedic surgery the lowest (10%) (ibid.; see also Association of American Medical Colleges 1996:803). Women's representation in medical faculties was much more skewed toward the lower ranks than was men's: 11 percent of women held the rank of full professor, 19 percent were associate professors, 50 percent were assistant professors, and 17 percent were instructors (Bickel 2000:10). Men's representation was much more balanced among the ranks: 31 percent were full professors, 25 percent were associate professors, 35 percent were assistant professors, and 8 percent were instructors.

The barriers to the higher-status positions still seem to be harder for women than for men to overcome. A cross-sectional survey of physicians on the faculty of U.S. medical schools who had been appointed between 1979 and 1981 examined the likelihood of having the rank of associate or full professor after a mean of eleven years of faculty service. The results showed that 59 percent of women and 83 percent of men had achieved the rank of associate or full professor. Only 5 percent of women but 23 percent of men had achieved the rank of full professor. There were several significant differences between men and women faculty. For example, women were less likely to have been allocated office space or dedicated laboratory space to begin their faculty careers with grant support, and to have protected time for research. Furthermore, men published significantly more

Table 3.5.    Women Physicians (%) by Type of Nonpatient Activity in the U.S. in 1970, 1980, and 1997

| Type of activity | Percentage female | | |
|---|---|---|---|
| | 1970 | 1980 | 1997 |
| Medical teaching | 11 | 14 | 22 |
| Administration | 7 | 10 | 15 |
| Research | 10 | 13 | 18 |
| Other | 11 | 14 | 20 |
| Total percentage of women | 9 | 12 | 18 |
| Total number of women | 2,956 | 4,737 | 7,946 |

Source:    Pasko and Seidman (1999:19, 31).

first-author publications: 27 percent of women published no first-author publications, but only 9 percent of men (Tesch et al. 1995:1023). And after productivity factors were adjusted for, women still remained less likely than men to be promoted (Tesch et al. 1995).

The same trend in academic publishing was documented in a study that covered full-time faculty in twenty-four U.S. medical schools (Barnett et al. 1998). The results showed that women faculty had published two-thirds as many articles as men, but this was not found to be accounted for by gender differences in career motivation. With respect to career motivation, men and women were similar in their views of the relative importance of intrinsic versus extrinsic career motivation (ibid.: 183).

A national study of the rates of advancement to the ranks of assistant, associate, and full professor for all U.S. medical school graduates from 1979 through 1993 and for all members of U.S. medical school faculties from 1979 through 1997 showed two diverse patterns (Nonnemaker 2000). First, women were significantly more likely than men to hold a faculty position at some point after graduation. Second, the proportion of women who advanced to the senior ranks of academic medicine was lower than that of their male colleagues, i.e., from assistant to associate, and from associate to full professor (ibid.:401)[2]. These findings suggest, on the one hand, that women medical students are a more select group than the male medical students at the start of their medical career. The findings indicate, on the other hand, the cumulative effect of promotion differentials and thus confirm the notion of the glass ceiling as the product of discrimination of women at each stage of their academic career (see Ferree and Purkayastha 2000).

The gendered structural barriers to a career in medicine are experienced early. A national survey of fourth-year U.S. medical students, conducted in 1996, showed little difference between male and female students in the feedback on performance in medical school (Bright, Duefield, and Stone 1998). But a number of indicators that tap perceptions of the career possibilities differed for male and female students. For example, fear of failure was experienced by 31 percent of the females, but by only 19 percent of the males. Furthermore, 60 percent of the females, but only 25 percent of the males reported that gender had an effect on their educational experience. And 30 percent of the females but only 7 percent of the males thought that they had to be twice as good as medical students of the opposite sex. Finding a mentor was hard for both male and female, but more females felt this to be a problem (27 percent) than males (19 percent). In more general terms, more women than men reported problems finding same-sex role models (18 percent versus 1 percent) and same-sex mentors (18 percent versus 3 percent). Moreover, in Everett Hughes's (1958) terms, the master status of the physician was male gendered: only 3 percent of the male medical students reported that they had been mistaken for a nonphysician while 92 percent of the female medical students had had this experience (Bright et al. 1998:684).

Another study of the interest in academic careers among first- and third-year residents in an U.S. medical school showed marked gender differences between the students as they proceed through their residence experience. For example, first-year women residents were slightly more inclined than the men (59 percent vs. 56 percent) to indicate that they anticipated an academic career, but this pattern had reversed by the third year: only 22 percent of the women expected at that point an academic career while 46 percent of the men still did. This response pattern is further supported by an increasing self-confidence among the men during the same period but a drop in self-confidence among the women: 82 percent of the first-year men residents and 70 percent of the women said they were self-confident, but three years later 89 percent of the men and only 65 percent of the women were. Similarly, there was no gender difference in the reported experience of stress by the first-year residents (about 70 percent experienced stress), but by the third year men's reporting of stress had dropped (59 percent) while women's had markedly risen (90 percent) (Leonard and Ellsbury 1996:503).

The studies referred to above all seem to have the same tacit message: Something happens to women during their training to become physicians that does not happen to the same extent to the men. The medical school still seems to be a gendered institution, where the premises for learning and advancing are based on masculinity as the norm. In the hierarchy of medicine, the process seems to be gendered so that fewer women than men reach top positions.

In the highest ranks of the profession there are still relatively few women. In 1998, 6 percent of the departmental chairs in U.S. medical schools were women. In 1999, in the 125 U.S. medical schools, only six women were deans. Compare this to the considerable advances made by women at the lower levels—associate and assistant dean (Bickel 2000:10). Similarly, the proportion of women in the House of Delegates of the American Medical Association grew from 5 percent in 1988 to 10 percent in 1994 (Kirschstein 1996). These figures indicate that women have began to enter the policymaking center of the profession.

## CONCLUSIONS

The review indicates that women physicians' advancement in U.S. medicine has been related to strategic transformations in medicine. Women entered medicine as practitioners in the age of cottage industry medicine, when a decentralized fee-for service medical market constituted the major medical mode of production. In this market, the gender system influenced medical practice so that women physicians' primary task was to take care of women and children.

American women entered medicine by a dual route: the private internal market and foreign-based coeducation in medicine. The unregulated medical market in mid–nineteenth century America enabled women to gain entry into medical schools and to practice medicine. A number of medical sects competed with the regular physicians in providing health care, but the market was segmented: while the regulars were mostly concentrated in urban areas, the sectarians catered mainly to the rural population. But this was the age of another segmentation, that by gender. Most of the first generation of women physicians were educated in separate medical colleges—either sectarian or women's—which put them in a marginalized position vis-á-vis the regular male physicians. This established a pattern of gender-segregated inclusion of women into U.S. medicine. Access to European medical education, based on scientific medicine, later to be emulated by U.S. mainstream male medicine, enabled the more career-oriented women not only to enter regular medicine but also to be better qualified than domestically trained men. As coeducational medical education became available to women, the proportion of women physicians stayed the same for almost fifty years, only to rise as an effort of affirmative action in the 1970s (Walsh 1977).

In the 1920s the preventive medicine perspective, valorized by women physicians during the era of social reform at the turn of the century, was challenged as U.S. medicine bifurcated into two professional paths due to the Flexner reform. U.S. medical schools standardized their education and the professionalization and specialization of medicine began to change the practice of U.S. physicians in the 1920s. At the same time public health became a new profession, and its practitioners were educated at the nation's new public health schools and worked in the state and county health departments that, because of public-health-related legislation, received new mandates and financing. For women physicians this meant no longer having the sole prerogative to the ethos of public health merely on account of their gender. On the other hand, as More (1999:156) has pointed out, ironically the Sheppard-Towner Act created a consciousness of children's health needs that opened a private market for such services. In this way, women found a new jurisdiction for their gender-specific skills in the emerging new specialty of pediatrics within mainstream medicine. As shown in this chapter, this specialty had the highest proportion (46 percent) of women physicians among all specialties in 1997.

In the 1930s, hospital medicine as a factorylike mode of production took off and medicine emerged as a scientific, hierarchically organized enterprise in which the medical profession exerted professional dominance over new, predominantly female health occupations, e.g., nurses and physician assistants. For women physicians, this medical mode of production was hard to enter because of its many gatekeeping mechanisms controlled by men. In the U.S. context, internships, residencies, peer referral systems, and hospital appointments were related to male mentors and to peer relations with male colleagues.

In the 1980s, a dramatic change in the mode of medical production began to take place in U.S. medicine, which shifted the economic and administrative control of medicine to forces outside the profession. The rise of corporate medicine has implied that U.S. physicians increasingly work as salaried employees in large group practices. This mode of production has influenced women physicians more than men: 56 percent of women physicians worked as employees in 1997, compared to 35 percent of men physicians (AMWA 2000:4).

Although employee status has been associated with the loss of power and autonomy of the medical profession, this "proletarianization" might eventually be advantageous for women. As Reskin and McBrier (2000:214) show, bureaucratizing personnel practices can promote open recruitment that undermines sex-based ascription and tends to increase women's share in, for example, managerial jobs. Similarly, bureaucratized practices can promote standardized job requirements and salaries and encourage more open recruitment practices.

The presentation of the career advancements of American women physicians during the twentieth century highlights four characteristics. First, the proportion of women in the profession remained almost constant between 1900 and 1970. As Table 3.2 indicates, the proportion of women in medicine in the United States remained the same (6 percent) from 1910 to 1950 and had reached 7 percent by 1970. Since 1970, a rapid increase in the number of women physicians can be discerned. In 1999, women physicians constituted 23 percent of U.S. physicians, and the figure is expected to rise to 29 percent in 2010. This projection is based on the entering cohort of women, who comprised 46 percent of the first-year medical students at allopathic medical schools in the United States in 1999–2000.

Second, women physicians in patient care are overrepresented in certain practice settings and medical specialties. For example, women physicians more often than men work as employees, and the range of specialties where most of them work is different. The most striking gender difference is the clustering of women in pediatrics and men in general surgery.

Third, due to their different practice and specialty profile, women physicians have a lower median income than men. Only 4 percent of physicians in the highest net-income quartile were women. In the lowest quartile, a third of the physicians were women.

Fourth, women are still underrepresented in nonpatient care: medical teaching, administration, and research. Work in these areas tends to be organized hierarchically, and women still are not well represented in the top positions in those hierarchies. Nevertheless, as the next chapter will show, women physicians in the United States are as well represented in nonpatient care as women physicians in Scandinavia are; and women in the United States are better represented in the top positions in academe than are women in Scandinavia.

## NOTES

1.  According to Starr (1982:99), in 1871 the sectarians represented roughly 13 percent of the total number of physicians (nearly 6,000 sectarians compared to 39,000 regulars), and in 1880, about 20 percent. In 1880, the sectarians ran 24 out of 100 medical schools. By 1900, the sectarians operated 34 medical schools, and the regulars 126. By the time of the Flexner report in 1910, the regulars operated 109 schools, and the sectarians 22 (*JAMA*, 1923:553).

2.  Similar disparities in faculty promotion to associate or full professor have been recorded between underrepresented minorities (African-American, Hispanic, Native-American) on medical school faculty and whites on medical school faculty (Fang, Moy, Colburn, and Hurley 2000).

# 4

# Conditions Influencing Women Physicians' Careers in Scandinavia

## WOMEN'S ENTRY INTO THE MEDICAL PROFESSION IN THE SCANDINAVIAN COUNTRIES

In her study of the first generation of women physicians in the Netherlands, Marland (1995:443) asks why Dutch women were so late and initially so slow to enter medicine. The same question can be posed for the Scandinavian countries. The first Dutch woman physician, Aletta Jacobs, qualified in medicine from the University of Groningen in 1878, the same year that the first woman, Rosina Heikel, got her medical degree and the right to practice medicine in Finland. Rosina Heikel was also the first woman to practice medicine in Scandinavia (Westermarck 1930). The early history of women's educational opportunities in the Scandinavian countries shows both similarities and divergences. A distinction will here be made between a Scandinavian model, represented by Sweden, Denmark, and Norway, and the Finnish pattern.

### The Scandinavian Path

The right for women to study and practice medicine in Sweden was achieved rather uneventfully. A (male) member of the peasant estate, C. J. Svensén, had submitted a motion to the 1859–1860 and 1862–1863 Diet of the four estates that women be granted the right to various offices, but the proposal met with little success. To further the cause, Svensén published in 1866 a booklet on women's rights ("Om qvinnans medborgerliga rättigheter"). He submitted a motion to the 1865–1866 Diet that women be granted the right to higher education and to pursue a doctoral degree in the humanities, the sciences, and medicine (Andreen [1956] 1988:9). This motion was approved and all medical faculties endorsed it in 1870, a measure that gave women the right to go to medical school (ibid.:10). The medical faculties recommended that men and women receive the same education and take the same examination. Hence, an explicit stance was taken approving coeducation and rejecting separatism or a special medical track for women. Three years later women were granted the right to study at all faculties at the University of Uppsala and Lund, except at the faculty of theology. The first women enrolled in medicine at the University of Uppsala in 1873, but it was not until 1888 that a woman, Karolina Widerström, got her medical degree. Before 1901, only eight women graduated in medicine in Sweden.[1] The academic career of women physicians was particularly slow. Women advanced faster in the humanities—the first woman to get a Ph.D. was Ellen Fries, who earned her doctorate in history at the University of Uppsala in 1883. From 1883 to 1911, altogether nineteen women got their doctorate in Sweden, but only two of them in medicine: Anna Stecksén in 1900, and Anna Dahlström in 1908 (Ohlander 1987).

In Denmark, women had been granted the right to study medicine at the University of Copenhagen in 1875, but the first woman to graduate— Nielsene Nielsen—did so ten years later (Schondel and Sørensen 1984). Nielsen's own accounts of her educational experiences and efforts to specialize in gynecology were of passive resistance from her own family and society to active discrimination by the key gatekeepers in her profession (Rosenbeck 1987). Also in Denmark, the first women to earn doctorates were in the field of history in 1893. Much later, in 1906, Eli Møller became the first woman to earn a doctorate in medicine.

In Norway, women were granted the right to attend the university in 1882, and in 1884 the right to earn an academic degree. This opened the opportunity for women to study medicine. The first woman to graduate was Marie Spångberg, in 1893 (Schiøtz and Nordhagen 1992). From 1893 to 1900, as many as eighteen women earned their medical degrees in Norway. In 1907, fourteen of these pioneering women were active private practitioners (ibid.:3789–90). From 1893 to 1920, women constituted 20 percent of the medical students in Norway (i.e., 59 out of 299), which was quite a high proportion for that time, in international terms (Blom 1987:9). The women came from the same socioeconomic groups as the men— urban, upper-middle class. Of the cohort, 54 percent of the women were to marry, as compared to 84 percent of the men; but as many as 75 percent of the married women remained active in the profession. One-third of the cohort were in private practice, and most clustered in gynecology, pediatrics, dermatology, pulmonary disease, and surgery. The higher echelons of the profession remained closed for women—of the 102 district physicians, only seven were women (Blom 1987, 1995). But also the academic career seemed hard to enter. The first Norwegian woman to gain a doctorate in medicine was Alexandra Ingier, in 1914; and the next was Inga Saeves, in 1916 (Schiøtz and Nordhagen 1992:3789). The pace was even slower during the subsequent decades. From 1920 to 1970, only three more women earned their doctorate in medicine: Kirsten Utheim Toverud in 1923, Eva Walaas in 1956, and Kirsten Osen in 1970 (Hovig 1993:2118).

The dates above highlight two features of women's entry into medicine in Sweden, Denmark, and Norway. First, the right to study medicine was given later than, for example, in Switzerland, France, and the Netherlands. Second, the humanities, especially history, provided the channel to a higher academic degree and career for women in Sweden and Denmark (and also Finland), while an academic career in medicine or the humanities seems to have been difficult for women to achieve in Norway. Furthermore, the biographical history of the pioneering women reveals that the decision to study medicine was not in the hands of profeminist professors of medicine as in St. Petersburg and Zurich but was considerably influenced by the perceived heroic character of the U.S. women physicians, whom the Scandinavian women strove to emulate. The first woman physicians in Sweden, in Norway, and in Denmark were each inspired by the news of the large number of women physicians practicing in the United States. In fact, the first Swedish woman to become a physician was Charlotte Yhlen, who went to the United States to study medicine at the Woman's Medical College of Pennsylvania in 1868. She received her U.S. medical degree in 1873 and returned to Sweden only to find that, with her foreign degree, she was not allowed to practice medicine. She enrolled in the medical school at Uppsala University but never began to study there. Instead, she returned to the United States and resumed her medical practice in Philadelphia (Andreen [1956] 1988:11).

The U.S. influence is also exemplified in the case of Norway: Four of Marie Spångberg's five brothers had moved to the United States and wrote to their sister in Norway about the many women doctors in the New World. The brothers not only encouraged, but more important, financed their sister's medical study back home in Norway (Schiøtz and Nordhagen 1992:3787). Similarly, in 1873 in Denmark, Nielsene Nielsen read in the newspaper about women physicians in the United States and decided to become a physician herself (Schondel and Sørensen 1984:14; Petersson 1998). She went to Copenhagen and did the matriculation examination in 1874. After that, she tried to find a mentor among foreign women physicians and finally managed to find a temporary one: the Swedish-born U.S. physician Charlotte Yhlen, described above, who visited Copenhagen for a scientific conference. She encouraged Nielsen to find a Danish male mentor, personified in the director of the City Hospital of Copenhagen, Dr. Fenger, who became committed to Nielsen's endeavor and urged the public authorities to grant her admission to the university. Fenger argued that it was important to educate women as physicians because, with "the development that the treatment for the female sex-specific diseases had enjoyed during recent years ... it also would be of great benefit for birthing, if there were women physicians" (Rosenbeck 1987:103).

In 1875, women were granted the right to study at the University of Copenhagen. During the deliberation, it was found out, ironically, that there had never been any explicit rule forbidding women to study at the university—it had just been taken for granted. This circumstance sparked a debate among the conservatives, who argued that restrictions in women's rights to higher education were justified by women's biological limitations (ibid.:104). Hence, in Denmark, as in so many other countries, women's right to study at the university is at the same time the tale of their right to medical education.

Although U.S. women physicians served as important role models for Scandinavian women, the first women medical students and women physicians were confronted with a conservative medical faculty and profession. In fact, the liberal and profeminist views of the medical faculty in St. Petersburg and in Zurich seem to have been an essential ingredient of the advancement of women's position in medical education there in the 1860s and the 1870s (Engel 1979; Bonner 1989). The anecdotal history from the Scandinavian countries does not paint a very favorable picture of the male medical professors in the late nineteenth century. When a proposal that women be admitted to medical study was presented to the National Assembly in Norway in 1882, the Assembly asked the "expert opinion" of the medical faculty. That faculty vehemently objected to the proposal, and its "expert opinion" reflects a very conservative outlook: "One gets the impression that women of this kind are somewhat absurd—there is no doubt that women are outside their natural domain." The reasons for women's lack of qualifications for medical work:

> The physician's calling demands . . . more than knowledge. It demands a certain mental and calm judgment, a firm character and will, a certain calm and balance of mind, which the woman often lacks or in any case can only with difficulties acquire. By contrast, the woman has other qualities, which make her particularly adapted to be the real nurse, a field to which she is already by nature assigned. (Schiøtz and Nordhagen 1992:3785)

In Denmark the medical faculty of the University of Copenhagen was hesitant to admit women to medical study but had grudgingly to consent: "when she submits to the same requirements as men." One of the professors Mathias Saxtorph, however, withheld his consent:

> The State in a way could be said to take indecency under its protection when it permits and arranges a prostitution system, but this is today considered a necessary evil. But women physicians could be called a totally unnecessary evil, which every Danish man certainly would like his country to be spared from. (Schondel and Sørensen 1984:15)

At least Professor Saxthorp was a man whose deeds were consistent with his thoughts. When the first woman physician, Nielsine Nielsen, was granted an internship at the municipal hospital in Copenhagen in 1885,

Saxthorp, then chief physician of the hospital, resigned in protest (Rosenbeck 1987:107).

Most of the pioneering Danish women physicians were confronted with active discrimination or passive resistance. For example, one of the first women medical students, Emilie Slamberg-Thrane, in 1898, was examined in gynecology by her male professor in a rather unusual way: during the whole examination he turned his back to her to indicate his misgivings about women's right to study medicine (Schondel and Sørensen 1884: 37).

## The Finnish Path

Finland has always been shaped by political and economic forces from the East and the West, and in medicine too. As a consequence of the Napoleonic wars in Europe, Finland was ceded by Sweden to Russia in 1809 and became an autonomous Grand Duchy within the Russian Empire. While the educational system in Finland was firmly founded on the Scandinavian system as part of its common history with Sweden, it was in the nineteenth century influenced to a considerable degree by its ties to Russia. This pertained not only to women's rights to enter higher education but to all academic matters. Two conditions related to the Russian rule influenced the academic system. First, formal decisions concerning the only university in Finland, the University of Helsinki, were not made by domestic authorities but by the Chancellor in St. Petersburg or by the tsar himself. Second, issues pertaining to women's status in the educational system in Finland were from the Russian authorities' side much influenced by women's rights to university study in Russia at the time (Engman 1987:35). Hence, as women aspired to entry into the university in Finland, Russian women had in the early 1860s been attending lectures at the university in St. Petersburg, and after 1872 general "higher courses for women" and a "women's medical course" were offered at the university (see also Chapter 5).

To enter the University of Helsinki, a candidate had to pass the matriculation examination, and courses preparing students for that were offered only at boys' gymnasiums. The first woman to pass the matriculation examination, in 1870, was the daughter of a wealthy Russian merchant in Helsinki; the second was Emma Irene Åström, the first woman admitted to the University of Helsinki, in 1872. Both women had been granted admission upon pleading for individual exemption from the general rules from the tsar—a system called dispensation. In 1873, two other women pleaded for exemption but were not granted admission. The next two women who applied, in 1885, were. By 1889, nineteen women had been given dispensation to study at the University of Helsinki. These nineteen were an exceptional lot—five of them earned a doctorate: three in medicine and two in history (Engman 1987, 1996:18).[2]

At the turn of the century, two other conditions came to have an effect on the number of women at the University of Helsinki—still the only university in Finland. First, the system of dispensation for women was abolished in 1901. Second, also in 1901, the first cohort of students with diplomas from coeducational schools graduated and was admitted to the university. The result of these new opportunity structures for women was that 733 women students were enrolled at the University of Helsinki that year.

In principle, then, women were given the right to attend university lectures in 1870 in Finland (at the same time as in Sweden); and by a special statute, on May 1, 1871, Tsar Alexander II granted women the right to study medicine at the University of Helsinki. The first woman to graduate in medicine was Rosina Heikel, who had won her medical degree in 1878 by asking the tsar's dispensation. As indicated earlier in this chapter, Rosina Heikel was the first to graduate and practice medicine in the Nordic countries (the next were Nielsene Nielsen in Denmark, in 1885; Karolina Widerström in Sweden, in 1888; and Marie Spångberg in Norway, in 1893). Like Rosina Heikel, the next women in Finland to get a medical degree, Ina Rosqvist and Karolina Eskelin, got their medical degrees in 1896 but they also had to ask the tsar for dispensation to graduate and get the right to practice. The authority to grant dispensation was given to the Senate in 1897. [Dispensation was a procedure used in Sweden, but more widely in Finland as a way of granting women access to education and offices in the public sector (Engman 1996:19).] From 1900 to 1910, thirteen women got their medical degrees (Parvio 1987).[3]

As women gained the right to study medicine, the medical profession had to grapple with the type of education provided to them: was it to be the kind of restricted education given, for example, in Russia at the time, or were they to be provided a general education? In 1873, the Finnish Medical Society assembled to debate these questions: "Whether there were any advantages to expect in health care in Finland from the fact that women had been granted the right to study at the medical faculty," and "Whether it is thereby necessary that their knowledge, as far as primary studies are concerned, is to be kept as high as for male students." The spirit among the male delegates was rather positive despite the negative slant of the question. Professor Wasastjerna opened the discussion:

> Among those fields in which a man's work could satisfactorily be replaced by a woman's, one hears from advocates for her expanded rights that, one of the foremost, physician's work is advanced as one of those for her talent the most natural and suitable.
>
> It cannot be denied that even if the woman does not to the same extent as a man possess some of a man's common characteristics that for the practicing physician are of great importance, such as cold bloodedness, capacity for calm deliberation, and basic critical reasoning, greater physical strength and

so on, she on the other hand possesses more than he does of tenderness and patience, a finer tact and nicer hand, which especially makes her suited to caring for her ill and suffering fellow human beings. [Finska Läkaresällskapet (FLS) 1875:31]

Although one conservative voice was heard, the other delegates reprimanded him for too traditional views. As another delegate was referring to both the practical benefit and justice of women's being permitted to enter, he mollified his colleagues by predicting the future gender segregation of medical practice: "I would envision that any real competition between male and female physicians will not take place, but that they will divide between them the great and ever expanding field of medicine" (ibid.:39).

In 1899, the same society assembled again around the issue of women physicians' access to various types of medical work and right to medical offices. The delegates of the society were quite liberal-minded and wanted to give more rights than the political decision-makers had proposed. But one of the delegates concluded that they were talking about exceptional conditions: "We have, however, to agree that it still is, and in all likelihood will so be at any time in the future, an exceptional case that a woman devote herself to a physician's work" (FLS 1900:60).

The picture that appears from reading the historical accounts on the attitudes of leading male physicians—professors of medicine and the medical societies—toward women's entry into the medical profession in the Scandinavian countries is that the initiators of women's emancipation were hardly in established medical circles during the period between 1870 and 1900. Instead, profeminist male politicians, spurred by women's rights advocates, were the ones endorsing women's rights to enter universities and the medical profession. On this matter, the attitudes of the medical elite seem to have been more conservative in Denmark and Norway than in Sweden and Finland. But until the first decades of this century, all four countries upheld restrictions on women physicians' right to hold state medical offices. In Norway, women got access to state offices in 1901, a law that was extended in 1912. In Denmark, state offices were opened to women in 1921. In Finland and Sweden, dispensation was practiced for a long time, enabling token numbers of women to hold public office, from which they were legally barred on the grounds of their gender. Finally, in 1925, in those two countries, women were granted the same right to state offices as men (Engman 1996:18).

## WOMEN PHYSICIANS IN SCANDINAVIAN MEDICINE IN THE TWENTIETH CENTURY

As was shown in the previous section, women in the Scandinavian countries entered the medical profession around the 1880s and 1890s. They were never trained in a separate medical track for women but were educated together with men and earned the same degree as men. All the same, the legislation to grant women the right to study medicine in 1870 in Sweden contained a disclaimer that denied women the right to occupy any public office in medicine. In the late nineteenth century, to be a public employee in a society that was still predominantly agrarian meant that the secure higher-income positions in medicine were reserved to men. The restriction was formally abolished in 1909 in Sweden but was still not implemented until 1925 (Andreen [1956] 1988:60). The restriction implied that a secondary labor market had been created for women, although token women were able to occupy public positions by applying for a dispensation.

A slow industrialization, a small middle class, and a dispersed rural population were conditions not conducive to the emergence of a large private market for health care in Norway, Finland, and Sweden. For the medical profession to become a modern profession and to expand its power basis in the age of the emerging industrialization of medicine and hospital medicine, the male segment of medicine rallied around the state and its public offices not only to maintain but to improve the economic status of the profession (Riska 1993). In this venture, women remained on the fringe of the development of medicine. For Norwegian, Swedish, and Finnish women physicians the structure of medicine was from the beginning dominated by the public sector. For example, in 1880, 90 percent of the physicians in Sweden were employed in the public sector. Although employed physicians declined to about 60 percent by the turn of the century, the proportion of private practitioners has remained the very small. The private physician has been more the exception than the rule (Bergstrand 1963:701).

The first generation of women physicians in the Scandinavian countries was well aware of the gender aspect of medical work, and most were involved in women's movements at the turn of the century, in some way or another. They worked for dress reform, for the regulation of prostitution, for social hygiene, and for public programs for improving the health of poor women and their children. Views about equal rights and gender equality characterized these endeavors.

As will be shown in the next section, since the early 1970s the primary care approach has been given a new emphasis in the public sector system. Through legislation most of the Scandinavian countries have given primary care a new structure and significance in the overall health care system—for example, a comprehensive publicly financed health service enacted in 1971 in Denmark, the Public Health Act in 1972 in Finland, the Municipal Health Services Act in 1982 in Norway, and the proposals for a family physician system in the 1990s in Sweden (Riska 1993; Twaddle 1999). This legislation created new jobs and opportunity structures for young physicians. Since a high proportion of young physicians have been women, the primary-care specialties of medicine have become more gender balanced, as this chapter will show.

## Developments in the Age of the Welfare State

In 1950, the proportion of women in the medical profession ranged from around 10 percent in Denmark, Norway, and Sweden to a high of 21 percent in Finland. There was almost no increase in the 1950s and 1960s, but since 1970 the proportion of women physicians has increased rapidly in all these countries (Table 4.1). By 2000, women physicians constituted about a third of the medical profession in Denmark and Norway, 39 percent in Sweden, and half of the physicians in Finland (Nordic Medical Associations 2000). These figures are expected to rise further, so that within twenty years the medical profession is likely to be either gender-balanced or female-dominated (Table 4.1). For example, in 1998, in Scandinavia a majority of the physicians under 30 years of age were women (65 percent in Finland, 61 percent in Denmark, 59 percent in Sweden, and 52 percent in Norway).

Although the proportion of women in the profession in the Scandinavian countries has increased, the gender segregation of medical work has tended to prevail. Women physicians are not evenly distributed within medical specialties or in the ranks of medicine. Women are more likely than men to work in specialties pertaining to the needs of children (pediatrics, child psychiatry) and the elderly (i.e., geriatrics) or involving routine (radiology) or subordinated work (anesthesiology). Women have in particular been able to advance in obstetrics and gynecology, a specialty that in Britain and the United States is still male-dominated and prestigious. Few women, by contrast, are found in surgery. In 2000, women constituted 14 percent of the surgeons in Finland, 10 and 11 percent in Denmark and Sweden, respectively, and only 5 percent in Norway (Table 4.2). As Table 3.4 indicates, in the United States in 1997, 9 percent of the surgeons were women.

The figures on chosen specialty during the past decade indicate a fairly stable pattern. This can be further confirmed by looking at the trend in Finland, where women currently constitute almost half of the profession. Between 1990 and 2000, in Finland, the proportion of women has increased even further in the female-dominated field of child psychiatry (e.g., to 78 percent in 1990 and 83 percent in 2000). An even more marked development has taken place in geriatrics, a new specialty where women already constituted 29 percent in 1990, and then climbed to 64 percent in 2000 [Finish Medical Association (FMA) 1990, 2000]. A somewhat different pattern, however, is to be found in the field of surgery. Here, the pace of change is much slower, yet progressive. In 2000, women constituted 14 percent of surgeons in Finland, compared with 6 percent in 1990, and 5 percent in

*Table 4.1.* Percentage of Women in the Medical Profession in
Denmark, Finland, Norway, and Sweden, 1950–2015

| Year | Denmark | Finland | Norway | Sweden |
|------|---------|---------|--------|--------|
| 1950 | 10 | 21 | 10 | 9 |
| 1960 | 11 | 22 | 10 | 13 |
| 1970 | 18 | 27 | 12 | 17 |
| 1980 | 20 | 33 | 15 | 25 |
| 1990 | 26 | 42 | 23 | 34 |
| 2000 | 35 | 50 | 31 | 39 |
| 2010 | 49 | 56 | 40 | 45 |
| 2015 | 55 | 60 | 45 | 48 |

*Source:*  Nordic Medical Associations (1996, 2000), Finnish Medical
Associations (2000), Norwegian Medical Association (2000),
Swedish Medical Association (2000), Haavio-Mannila (1975:5),
Hofoss et al. (1983:37) statistics provided by the Danish Medical
Association.

1985. In the other Scandinavian countries, the proportions were even
smaller (Table 4.2).

Surgery seems to be an anomaly among medical specialties, suggesting
that little has changed in the organization of this kind of medical work.
Surgery is still performed within the hierarchical and closed structure of
hospital medicine. Changes in health care or health policies have had little
impact on surgery and no new opportunity structures have emerged as
they have in many primary-care specialties. Interviews with female surgeons in Norway (Dahle 1994; Nore 1993; Gjerberg and Hofoss 1998), Finland (Riska and Wegar 1993b), and Sweden (Einarsdottir 1997, 1999;
Lindgren 1999) have documented that the male-gendered medical culture
of surgery forms more of an obstacle to women physicians' entrance into
and advancement in surgery than does their own capacity to perform the
actual work (this aspect will be discussed further in Chapter 6). A Norwegian study showed that women were as likely as men to start their career
in surgery but that a far higher proportion of men (48 percent) than
women (20 percent) completed their specialist training in general surgery
or other surgical fields (Gjerberg 2001b).

In the hierarchy of medicine in Scandinavia, women are also still underrepresented in higher administrative positions (Korremann 1994). The distribution of women physicians in various sectors of the health care system
in Finland may be indicative of the prevailing trend. As Table 4.3 shows,
they have gained in all areas, but the internal pattern has remained.

A majority of primary care physicians in the public sector in Finland are
women. For example, in 2000, they constituted 58 percent of the physicians

Table 4.2. Percentage of Women in Selected Specialties in Denmark, Finland, Norway, and Sweden in 2000

| Specialty | Denmark | Finland | Norway | Sweden |
|---|---|---|---|---|
| Anesthesiology | 23 | 39 | 17 | 26 |
| Child and adolescent psychiatry | 56 | 83 | 61 | 59 |
| Dermatology and venereology | 38 | 66 | 28 | 59 |
| General practice | 30 | 46 | 21 | 40 |
| Geriatrics | 35 | 64 | 31 | 60 |
| Internal medicine | 17 | 34 | 13 | 29 |
| Pathology | 41 | 28 | 28 | 27 |
| Pediatrics | 42 | 58 | 26 | 41 |
| Psychiatry | 39 | 51 | 32 | 47 |
| Obstetrics and gynecology | 36 | 54 | 32 | 49 |
| Ophthalmology | 23 | 46 | 20 | 50 |
| Surgery | 10 | 14 | 5 | 11 |
| Women as a percentage of all specialists | 27 | 42 | 21 | 35 |

Source: Finnish Medical Association (2000), Norwegian Medical Association (2000), Swedish Medical Association (2000), statistics provided by the Danish Medical Association.

working at municipal health centers, which are the major entry points to the primary-care system at the local level. No specialization is required of physicians working at this level, which may be interpreted both as a reason for and consequence of women's working in this type of setting. The gender difference in the extent to which women and men physicians tend to specialize has become more accentuated over the past twenty-five years. In 1990, 33 percent of the women physicians in Finland were specialists, compared to 44 percent in 2000, while among men the proportion of specialists increased from 55 percent in 1990 to 57 percent in 2000. The same trend has been documented in Norway: For example, in 1972, 28 percent of the women and 40 percent of the men were specialists, and in 1998, 41 percent of the women and 66 percent of the men (Gjerberg 2001a:334–36). On the other hand, a majority of the Finnish physicians under the age of thirty years (67 percent in Finland in 2000) are women who are currently residents, and thus the so-called representational lag of women among specialists will even out in the future. This was confirmed in the foregoing Norwegian study, which showed that the younger cohort of women physicians, as compared to an older one, specialized as often as men in 1997 (almost 80 percent) (ibid.:336).

These figures indicate two ongoing processes. Women may today be less inclined to specialize because there is, since the Public Health Act of 1972 in Finland, a new opportunity—the health center physician posts in the

*Table 4.3.* Distribution (%) of Physicians in Finland by Main Employment in 2000, and Percentage of Females in the Main Areas in 1990 and 2000

| Main employment | All physicians 2000 | Percentage of females in the area | |
|---|---|---|---|
| | | 1990 | 2000 |
| Hospitals | 37 | 37 | 46 |
| Health centers | 20 | 54 | 58 |
| Ambulatory clinics | 3 | 53 | 64 |
| Occupational health | 3 | 38 | 47 |
| Private practice | 6 | 50 | 50 |
| Teaching, research | 7 | 25 | 42 |
| Administration | 4 | 29 | 39 |
| Not practicing | 16 | 42 | 46 |
| unemployed | 1 | | |
| retired | 12 | | |
| other | 3 | | |
| Abroad | 5 | | |
| Total (%) | 100 | 42 | 50 |
| N | 18,590 | 5,780 | 8,928 |

*Source:* Finnish Medical Association (1990, 2000).

public sector—that does not require specialization. Similarly, the Municipal Health Services Act enacted a decade later in Norway also offered a new opportunity structure, but establishing at the same time public health and general practice as specialties required for physicians practicing in those settings (ibid.:340). On the other hand, interview data tend to suggest that the health center setting is a flat organizational structure, which provides women physicians more professional autonomy in their work than the hierarchical structure of the hospital. Furthermore, work at a health center is characterized by regular hours, in contrast to work at a hospital—a fact that allows women to combine professional and family life. Further support for this is found in a Finnish study (Riska and Wegar 1995), a British study (Brooks 1998) and a Norwegian study (Gjerberg 2001a:340) on reasons given by women physicians for the choice of general practice.

Ironically, part-time work has been a political issue but one that has mainly concerned men who have wanted to have a subsidiary practice, generally in the private sector, in addition to their main employment in the public sector. This issue of subsidiary practice has been debated in Swedish medicine over the past fifty years as an effort by the Social Democratic Party to curtail private practice (Garpenby 1989; Twaddle 1999). More men than women have practiced privately. A survey of the work conditions of physicians in Finland in 1997 showed that 59 percent of the men and 31 percent of the women had a subsidiary private practice (and of those, men for 6.7 hours a week and women for 5.2 hours). Pay for the subsidiary work provided 23 percent of the men's and 19 percent of the women's income (Töyry et al. 2001).

Part-time practice or a "mommy track" as an option for women physicians has not been seriously debated in Scandinavian medicine. The only time part-time work for physicians was discussed, for example, in Finland was during the time of high unemployment (7 percent) among them in the early 1990s. Then the Finnish Medical Association appealed to the older generation of physicians to retire early or to work part-time in order to leave their jobs in the public sector to the new medical school graduates (a majority of whom were women) (Riska 1995; Löyttyniemi 2000).

Only a small proportion of all physicians in Finland and Sweden (6 percent and 7 percent in 2000, respectively) work in the private sector. In Finland this is a gender-balanced sector. Private physicians work mainly in the metropolitan area of Helsinki and are specialists, clustered mainly in ophthalmology, obstetrics and gynecology, and psychiatry (FMA 1996). In these areas, between 46 and 54 percent are women (Table 4.2 ).

Table 4.3 shows that Finnish women physicians have advanced in two important areas—administration, and teaching and research. Today, women constitute about 40 percent of those working in these areas, compared to one-fourth to almost a third respectively a decade ago. The advancement of women in these areas is worth noting for two reasons. First, these areas have been identified as the male-dominated bastions, in which the in-group and mentor system has apparently prevented women from advancing (Lorber 1984, 1993).

Second, those who work in teaching, medical research, and administration determine the content and priorities of future medicine. If more women work in these areas, it could at least be argued that they will have some impact on the content of medical knowledge and medical education in the future. Nevertheless, close examination shows that women still occupy the lower positions in these fields in Scandinavia and are not equally represented with men in the top positions (Korremann 1994:40). For example in Finland in 1996, only 20 percent of the chief physicians at hospitals and 30 percent of the chief physicians at municipal health centers were women (FMA 1996). In 1996, women comprised an even smaller percentage of professors of medicine (19 percent) in Finland than in Norway (13 percent) and in Denmark (8 percent). The figures are even lower in Sweden, where in 1996 only 6 percent of the professors in medical schools were women (Ståhle 1998:81). Figures for the lower academic positions have not been much more promising: women constitute 44 percent of bio-medical Ph.D.s, but they hold a mere 25 percent of the postdoctoral positions, a discrepancy that has sparked a lot of debate about gender and research funding in Sweden (Wennerås and Wold 1997:341). The Finnish figures are somewhat more promising.[4] Among postdoctoral researchers supported by the Academy of Finland, which is the Finnish National Science Foundation, in 1999 women constituted 41 percent of researchers in the health sciences but 14 percent of researchers in the natural sciences. The social sciences and humanities had gender-balanced proportions among the postdoctoral researchers.

Following Kanter's (1977) "token" argument, as long as women's representation in the top administrative and academic positions is low, women might not have much real influence in setting the guidelines for future practice of medicine or medical knowledge. Yet, there are individual women in academic medicine who have managed to challenge and to have an impact on health care delivery and medical knowledge concerning women. Nevertheless, these women are not part of a movement of academic women physicians in the same way as, for example, those acting within the American Women's Medical Association. Although there were national branches of the International Women's Medical Association in the Scandinavian countries in the past—for example, the Finnish Women Physicians' Association (Suomen Naislääkäriyhdistys 1987; Parvio 1987) in Finland—the collective consciousness that characterized these pioneering women has largely been lost with the integrationist endeavors of the later generation of Scandinavian women physicians.

The figures above on women's position in medical work in the Scandinavian countries all suggest a progressive trend despite a pattern of gender segregation. Furthermore, the data show, on average, an increase of women's representation in academic medicine but lend also support to the metaphor of the existence of a glass ceiling that hampers women's advancement above a certain rank in medicine (Lorber 1993, 2000a; Ferree and Purkayastha 2000). The effects of this glass ceiling seems to be stronger in Scandinavia than in the United States, since the proportions of women in academic medicine in Scandinavia are much lower than the figures for women in U.S. medicine.

## CONCLUSIONS

This chapter has examined women's entry into and later careers in medicine in the Scandinavian countries. The review indicates that women's advancement in medicine has been related to strategic transformations in medicine. In the United States, women entered medicine as practitioners in the age of cottage industry medicine, when a decentralized fee-for-service medical market constituted the major mode of medical production. In this market, the gender system influenced medical practice so that women physicians' primary task was to take care of women and children. Women and children were also the major constituency of the pioneering physicians in Scandinavia. But Scandinavian women were slow to enter medicine despite the ideology of gender equality. The proportion of women in the medical profession remained low during the first decades of the twentieth century.

In the 1920s and 1930s, hospital medicine in a factorylike mode of production took off and medicine emerged as a scientific, hierarchically organized enterprise. For women physicians, this mode of medical production was hard to enter because of its many gatekeeping mechanisms controlled by men. As shown in Chapter 3, in the U.S. context, internships, peer referral systems, and hospital appointments were related to male mentors and to peer relations with male colleagues. While the same factors were not insignificant in the Scandinavian context, the fact that most hospitals were part of the public sector became an additional obstacle. Women remained in the private sector of medicine since they were legally barred from most medical offices in the public sector. Furthermore, hospital medicine was from the beginning part of the public sector, where the positions were salaried. During that time, positions in the public sector were high status and well-paid and remained in the hands of men. In a health care system with a marginal private market, the hospital salary provided not only a secure full-time income but also an opportunity to refer patients to a part-time private specialty practice—a system that, for example, the social-democratic government in Sweden has tried since the 1950s to curb (Garpenby 1989, 1999; Twaddle 1999).

During the age of the welfare state, the medical profession has become one of the "welfare state occupations" because its work, professional position, and legitimacy derive from their function in the welfare state (Elzinga 1990:162; Evertsson 2000). The welfare-state occupations have been delegated the implementation of the goals and obligations that the state has been given, based on the principle of universal access of services and equity.

In the 1980s, the mode of production in U.S. medicine began to change dramatically, shifting the economic and administrative control of medicine to forces outside the profession. The rise of corporate medicine has implied that more and more U.S. physicians work as salaried employees in large group practices. The salaried status of the Scandinavian physicians has been a dominant pattern of practice during most of the twentieth century. Although the profession in Scandinavia has been characterized by the physicians' being employees, a comparable rapid "feminization" of the medical profession has not taken place in Scandinavia as it had in Soviet medicine (see Chapter 5).

A change could be witnessed in the labor-market position of physicians in Sweden and Finland in the 1990s. Financing and decision-making on health policies and uses of health care resources were decentralized in Sweden and Finland in the 1990s, with authority moving from the state to local government. The recession hitting Finland in the early 1990s and Sweden in the late 1990s implied falling tax revenues. This has meant a need to cut public spending due to restricted local tax resources. Despite this trend, there is still a commitment to universal access and to maintaining a strong public system, although a number of "market mechanisms" have been introduced to make the public system more cost-efficient (Twaddle 1999).

During the recession in the 1990s, a position as a salaried physician in the local public sector health care system was difficult to get for a newly graduated physician in Finland or Sweden (Riska 1995; Löyttyniemi 2000). Public health and primary care are still prioritized by public authorities, and the areas of medicine where women are practicing are officially endorsed as the ones implementing the goals of equity promoted by the welfare state. At the same time, the constraints of public financing at the local level have hit the primary care areas hardest, and these areas tend to be female-dominated.

## NOTES

1. The other seven women were Hedda Andersson (1892), Maria Folkesson (1896), Ellen Sandelin (1897), Sofia Holmgren (1898), Anna Dahlström (1899), Elin Beckman (1901), and Matilda Lundberg (1901) (Andreen [1956] 1988:63).

2. According to Tuve (1984:34, 59), among the first students to attend the University of Helsinki in 1870 were two Russian women—Adelaide Lukanina and Anna Shabanova—who were to be leading figures among the first generation of Russian women physicians. The former went to Zurich to study in 1871 and then to the United States, and the latter returned in 1873 to St. Petersburg to continue her studies in the special women's medical program. I have, however, not been able to verify this information in any of the Finnish sources on the pioneering women enrolled at the University of Helsinki in 1870–1873.

3. The thirteen women who graduated in medicine in Finland from 1900 to 1910 were Elin Augusta Elmgren (1900), Naema Ericson (1900), Alfhild Elisabeth Heideman (1900), Ellen Maria Ahlqvist (1901), Augusta Elisabeth Backman (1904), Viva Lagerborg (1904), Anna Elisabeth Wikander (1904), Martha Maria Prytz-Brander (1905), Eva Piispanen (2907), Laimi Leidenius (1908), Selma Rainio (Lilius) (1908), Helmi Heikinheimo (1910), and Suoma Helena Loimaranta (1910) (Parvio 1987:18–19).

4. Among the European Union countries, Finland had the highest proportion of women professors (18 percent) in 1998, followed by Portugal (17 percent) and France (14 percent), while Sweden and Norway (11 percent) and Denmark (7 percent) had considerably lower proportions. The figure for 1998 given for the United States was 14 percent (Simons and Featherstone 2000:1101).

# 5

## Women Physicians in Russia and the Soviet Union

### FOUR PHASES IN THE EARLY EDUCATION OF RUSSIAN WOMEN PHYSICIANS

I am as furious as a chained watchdog; I have twenty-three villages, yet up to the present I haven't gotten as much as one cot and, probably, never will get that assistant who was promised me at the Medical Council. I drive from factory to factory begging, as if for alms, for premises to shelter my future patients. From morning to evening I am driving about, and I am already exhausted, even though cholera hasn't appeared yet.

—Anton Chekhov in a letter on July 22, 1892, to N. M. Lintvareva from Melikhovo, where he served as a zemstvo physician

For Russian women before 1900 the opportunities to study medicine can be divided into four phases. The first phase was from 1859 to 1864, a period characterized by political radicalism among students. This was a period when the upper- and middle-class youth in St. Petersburg and Moscow revolted against social institutions standing for traditionalism, foremost the patriarchal family and its values, and extolled services to "the people," the poor in the countryside. This latter common cause peaked from 1874 onward in a populist and radical movement among the students, a movement that became the seedbed for the prerevolutionary radicals (Engel 1979:402; Stites 1990:138–54).

In Russia, medical education was patterned after the European model: It was a university- and basic-science-based education. In 1861, several women applied for admission to study medicine, and while the state bureaucracy pondered the matter, women began to attend classes at the Medical Surgical Academy at St. Petersburg encouraged by the (male) professors of chemistry, physiology, and anatomy. Nevertheless, politically conservative circles began to fear the radicalism of the student movement, and the major target of the criticism was women students, whose mere presence in the movement epitomized the attack on patriarchal family values. In an effort to suppress student radicalism, especially among the

73

women, women were barred from universities in 1863 and from the Medical Surgical Academy in 1864 (Engel 1979). A number of women whose medical education was cut short in this way resumed their medical studies in Switzerland at the University of Zurich.

Hence the period from 1864 to 1872 constitutes the second phase among the opportunities available for Russian women to study medicine before 1900, although foreign based and used by young women from an affluent background—daughters of the nobility, civil servants, and Jewish merchants (ibid.:398). One of the first to transfer her studies from St. Petersburg to Zurich was Maria Knjaznina, the first woman to be permitted to enroll in medical courses at the University of Zurich in 1864. A year later Nadezhda Suslova began her studies and, in 1867, was the first woman to receive a medical degree from Zurich (Tuve 1984; Bonner 1989). At her dissertation defense, Edmund Rose, the professor of surgery of the medical faculty not only praised Suslova's achievement but linked her endeavor to a much broader social cause, saying (Tuve 1984:21):

> Soon we are coming to the end of slavery of women, and soon we will have the practical emancipation of women in every country and with it the right to work.

Upon her return to Russia in 1868, Suslova opened a private practice in St. Petersburg.

In the fall of 1871, twenty-one Russian women had enrolled in the medical faculty in Zurich, and during the next two years, sixty-four other women began to study medicine there (Engel 1979:408; Tuve 1984:24). Between 1864 and 1874, 120 Russian women (twice the number of men) had attended the University of Zurich, and 71 percent or eighty-five of them were in medicine (Stites 1990:84, 131). In 1873, the Russian government prohibited Russian students from enrolling for study in Zurich as it feared that the growing radicalism in the Russian student colony would spread back to the students in St. Petersburg. This prohibition was directed especially to the women students, who were ordered to leave Zurich with the message that future opportunities for education and employment in Russia would be suspended (Edmondson 1984:18).

The third phase of medical education for Russian women was between 1872 and 1887, when medical courses again became available to women in Russia. At the end of the 1860s, there were strong voices for offering higher education to women, and a plan for providing special medical courses for women was presented to the Ministry of Education (Tuve 1984:60). The Ministry of Education initiated evening lecture courses for women in 1869. In 1872, "higher courses for women" were provided in Moscow. During the first year, sixty-five women enrolled, to be followed by 160 women a year until this educational opportunity for women was closed in 1886. Until then similar opportunities had also been provided women in Kazan and Kiev (Stites 1990:81–82).

In the late 1860s, women began again to attend lectures, laboratories, and anatomy theatres at the male-dominated Medical Surgical Academy in St. Petersburg and were encouraged by the male professors at the medical faculty. A public appeal to women's caring skills as a rationale for permitting women to study medicine gradually softened the conservative bureaucrats. In 1872, a special track for women to be trained as midwives in a four-year medical program titled "Course for Professional Midwives" was established. In 1876, this program was extended to five years and retitled "Women's Medical Course." By now, women received the same education as men although by means of a segregated medical track. The first eighty-nine women admitted to the all-women program were taught by the (male) faculty of the Medical Surgical Academy in St. Petersburg. The women in this program differed in their social background from those women who at that time were studying medicine in Zurich. The women in the Women's Medical Course were the daughters of civil servants, military officers, and members of various professions (Engel 1979:398), while the women who had studied in Zurich had a more affluent background, e.g., the nobility.

As the first cohort of women graduated, they found out that they were restricted in their practice to treating women and children. An opportunity to challenge the restrictions imposed on women came: the whole cohort of twenty-five who graduated in 1877 went to serve in the Turkish war, twenty of them as medical assistants with the army, and five with the Red Cross (Stites 1990:86). Other sources provide even higher figures. According to Engel (1979:406), forty women medical graduates and twelve students served in the Turkish war from 1877 to 1978. Women independently did surgical operations and doctors' work. Upon their return from the war, not only were they praised and decorated but the tsar officially also granted that a woman medical graduate from then onwards be known as a "woman physician" (*Zhenskii Varch*) instead of "professional midwife" (*Uchenye Akusherki*) (Stites 1990:86; Engel 1979:414). Women physicians' rights were gradually extended, and by 1883 they gained formal recognition by their male colleagues as they were included in the medical register of physicians (Tuve 1984:67).

Altogether 691 women graduated from the Women's Medical Course, which was totally gender-segregated.[1] The admittance of new women medical students stopped in 1882, and the program was officially closed in 1887 (Engel 1979:408). Women again headed abroad. In 1894 and 1895, 151 of the 195 foreign women studying medicine at the University of Paris were Russian (Tuve 1984:108).

The fourth phase in the opportunities available for Russian women to study medicine began in 1895, when Tsar Nicolas II approved the founding of the Women's Medical Institute in St. Petersburg. Gender-segregated, it opened its doors in 1897. An ambitious undertaking, the new institute was designed for up to 1,500 students. By 1917, 2,804 women had graduated from it (Tuve 1984:110–14). Women's presence in the medical profession became even more pronounced during the prerevolutionary years. As Rayan (1989:37) points out, although the total number of civilian doctors remained almost the same during the years from 1914 to 1917 (24,031 in 1914 and 24,000 in 1917), the number of women doctors almost doubled (from 2,322 to 4,000 in the same period).

After the revolution in 1917, the institute, renamed the Leningrad Medical Institute, became coeducational. Nevertheless, it remained female-dominated, as the following figures amply tell: from 1917 to 1927, 4,669 women and 492 men graduated from it (Tuve 1984:118).

## THE DEMISE OF ZEMSTVO MEDICINE AND THE RISE OF SOVIET MEDICINE: THE FEMINIZATION OF MEDICAL WORK

The concept of "zemstvo medicine" is surrounded by a certain halo in the history of prerevolutionary Russian medicine. This institution has been bestowed with a set of values—a public ethos—that historians have suggested far exceeds its real significance in providing medical care and having an impact on the health of the Russian population. In his review of the fate of zemstvo medicine, Hutchinson suggests that there always was "more morality than medicine at the heart of the enterprise" (1990:22). The mythic elements of zemstvo medicine derive from the historical conditions surrounding its inception. This institution of medicine was part of the reforms introduced by the tsarist government, embodied as Alexander II, as a consequence of the 1861 Emancipation Proclamation, which freed the serfs. District assemblies—zemstvos—were established in 1864. The zemstvo was a form of local self-government that, through local tax revenues, was given the responsibility for the provision of public welfare, roads, education, medical care, and public health in rural Russia (Field 1957:1; Tuve 1984:2). But perhaps more importantly it was a historic endeavor that became pregnant with hopes for a real and democratic change of Russian society, although instituted by the tsarist government itself. Its public ethos was adopted and amplified by the urban-based intellectual and youth movement in the 1860s that propagated "services to the people." Among these populists were a number of physicians who, guided by progressive ideas, wanted to improve the living and health conditions of the local population through their professional services and by working for social reforms.

In the area of health care, the zemstvo employed a district physician, who provided medical care free of charge to the populace. This system was never really able to meet the health needs of the peasants because of lack of funds to employ physicians as well as because of the physicians' hesitancy to take up practice in remote and poor rural areas. As Mark Field (1957:5) observes in his classic on the Soviet physician, by 1892, out of more than 12,000 physicians, only 15 percent were zemstvo physicians. The figures improved but slowly: in 1870, there were 610 zemstvo physicians while there were 1,350 dispensaries with feldshers—a kind of physician assistant—available to the peasants, figures that by 1910 had risen to 3,100 zemstvo physicians and 2,620 feldsher dispensaries (ibid.:3; Ramer 1990:123). As Field notes, zemstvo medicine was, however, not a universal, nationwide medical care system but one that varied from one area to the other. A later observer of Soviet medicine (Navarro 1977:9) has argued that one of the novel features that zemstvo medicine instituted in Russia was a principle of regionalization of health care: the dispensaries in the zemstvos provided primary care, and specialized care was offered by the provincial hospital.

By 1917, the institution of zemstvo medicine had become an obsolete ideological hybrid in two ways. On the one hand, it represented an ideological continuity of public medicine that the new regime wanted to extend to the whole society. On the other hand, it represented a historic remnant of the tsarist era and services to a social class—the peasants—that had a low priority in the hierarchy of values of the new social order. So did another institution—the insurance movement for health care—which had been advanced by the trade union branch of the working-class movement. After the revolution, an insurance system administered by the working class and its unions was transformed into a universal and centralized national system—historically referred to as Soviet medicine (Ewing 1990:70–73).

The foundation of the Commissariat of Health (*Narodnii kommissariat zdravookhranenia*) in 1918 can be said to have constituted the demarcation line between the decentralized system of zemstvo medicine as well as the workers' insurance movement and the gradual emergence of Soviet medicine—a unified and centralized health care system that provided universally available health care services (Weissman 1990; Field 1957:17). The Commissariat of Health began to implement the goals and the structure of health care envisioned by the new regime. However, the geographical maldistribution of physicians continued. Both men and women were drawn to more lucrative private practices in the cities, notably Moscow and St. Petersburg. This pattern did not change with the revolution. In 1921, 45 percent of the rural posts were vacant; and in 1924 still 80 percent of all physicians resided in large cities, more than one-third in Moscow and Leningrad alone (Weissman 1990:114). By 1929 the figures had become even worse, with only 14 percent of physicians practicing in the countryside, and 8.5 percent preferring to be unemployed than to go to remote rural areas (Ramer 1990:135). Furthermore, during the era of the New Economic Policy (NEP) in the 1920s, the private practice of medicine continued, and survived well into the 1930s. It has been estimated that in 1930, 5 percent of the hospitals and 6 percent of the outpatient clinics were private; and as many as 18 percent of the physicians in Moscow were in private practice (Davis 1990:161).

Within the new health care system—Soviet medicine—an emphasis on new types of medical knowledge and a leveling off of medical workers emerged. In terms of the production and focus of medical knowledge, the history of Soviet medicine can be divided into two phases (Barr and Field 1996:307). The first phase can be identified with the 1920s, when the new regime held to a rigid Marxist interpretation of the etiology of illness: Illness was a product of the social and working conditions of capitalist society, and thus most social problems and diseases would wither away with the advent of socialism. The ideological focus of medicine was on prevention and a concomitant deemphasis of scientific and clinical medicine. However, resources and structures for developing a preventive approach never materialized, although a system of maternity and child care was initiated (Tuve 1984:116; Barr and Schmid 1996).

The second phase began with the industrialization of Soviet society as the NEP was launched and implemented in the early 1930s. During this phase, the production of new medical knowledge centered around industrial workers and their health problems. New types of specialization emerged to address the health needs of the "proletariat" or for those holding posts in the health administration, all new areas that became more prestigious than work as a state-employed general practitioner (yet there was no school of public health).

During the 1920s, the traditional characteristics of the medical profession were slowly dismantled. The medical profession lost its professional autonomy, control over its knowledge base, education, recruitment of new members, and its conditions of work and remuneration.

Medical education was almost totally removed from the universities in the 1930s, and transferred to vocational institutes supervised by the Ministry of Health (Barr and Schmid 1996). The medical programs gave a broad general training, and no opportunities for postgraduate education were provided. Ironically, Soviet medicine acquired two features related to U.S. preindustrial and "postindustrial" medicine. As Barr and Schmid (ibid.:142) in their examination of the features of medical education in the former Soviet Union point out, by the 1930s medical education in the Soviet

Union had reverted to features resembling pre-Flexnerian medical education in the United States. Because of the Flexner report of 1910 U.S. medical education began to emulate the science- and university-based medical and clinical programs developed in Europe at the time, and the era of free-standing medical institutes had ended by the latter part of the 1910s. By contrast, the Russian revolution during the same decade dramatically changed Russian medical education from university- to institute-based vocational education. Furthermore, Soviet medicine became the kind of "proletarianized" work that McKinlay and his colleagues (McKinlay and Arches 1985) envisioned as characterizing the U.S. medical profession with the advent of corporate medicine in the 1980s.

The abolishment of the professional dominance of the medical profession meant that the physician became one of the many employees among different groups of medical workers (Solomon 1990; Barr and Schmid 1996). Although there was a functional differentiation among the various groups of medical workers, there were no major salary differentials or hierarchies based on importance of work (Rayan 1989:20). Furthermore, the focus of the economy on industrial production devalued the work done in the social and health sector and transformed the social and gender composition of the physician workforce. Because of the special emphasis of the state-prioritized economic policy (i.e., NEP), medicine was considered a nonproductive activity and was less valued than engineering and vocational education preparing for work in industrial production. For example, the quotas for admission of students of proletarian origin were lower (60 percent) for medical schools than for technical and agricultural schools (75 percent) (Field 1957:67). Thus, male students and male workers flocked to the both financially and prestigiously more highly valorized jobs in industrial production. In this way, women and so-called nonproletarian elements came to be overrepresented in medicine, which was an area of secondary importance in status and remuneration in the overall hierarchy of work in Soviet society (Field 1957:67–69; Tuve 1984:125; Navarro 1977:48; Rayan 1989:38). Reskin and Roos (1990) have called this development of the labor market "double queueing," a process whereby a ranking of workers and of jobs has a gendered character. According to Reskin and Roos (ibid.:30), the labor markets can be conceptualized as consisting of labor queues and job queues. In this selection process society grants men first choice of jobs, and men select the most attractive, highly ranked jobs.

Since the 1920s, the physician workforce in the Soviet Union gradually began to have a female-dominated composition. Internationally, the proportion of women was rather high as early as the beginning of the twentieth century (Table 5.1). Its subsequent rise to constitute a majority twenty years later was, however, due to reasons different from those prevalent

*Table 5.1.* Women Physicians as a Percentage
of All Doctors in Russia/Soviet Union,
1910–1990

| Year | Percentage of women physicians |
|------|--------------------------------|
| 1910[a] | 10 |
| 1920 | n.a. |
| 1930 | 45 |
| 1940 | 62 |
| 1950 | 77 |
| 1960 | 76 |
| 1970 | 72 |
| 1980 | 69 |
| 1990 | 69 |

*Source:* Field (1967:118, 1975:462), Rayan (1989:41).
[a]Data are from 1913.    n.a., data not available.

when women entered medicine in the early 1870s. As shown earlier in this
chapter, the early entry of women into Russian medicine was related to the
gender-segregated track instituted in state-supported medical education.
Women were not only trained separately from men but they were also
expected to pursue different medical careers—to provide medical care for
women and children. This was a pattern of gender-segregated inclusion of
women into medicine.

While almost half of the first generation of women physicians entered
zemstvo medicine, the later cohorts did not. For many women physicians,
to live in a city and be unemployed was for family reasons preferable to
moving to the country (Weissman 1990:114). In Soviet medicine this pattern prevailed even later. It has been estimated that in the 1920s 70 percent
of unemployed physicians were women (Ramer 1990:135–37).

By 1950, the medical profession was a solidly female profession, with 77
percent of its practitioners being women (Table 5.1). In his classic on the
Soviet physician, Mark Field reflects on the doctors' living conditions,
work satisfaction, importance attached to the services rendered, status of
the profession, and its gender composition, and finds that they "resemble
to a striking degree those of the elementary and secondary school teacher
in the United States" (1957:26).

Another, but later, observer of Soviet medicine, Navarro (1977:79–80),
explicitly raises the issue of women as providers of health services in the
Soviet Union and addresses the "feminization" of Soviet medicine. He
asks, like many before and after him, whether the low prestige of the work
of the physician in Soviet medicine is due to the predominance of women,

and he is at least inclined to answer in the negative. The feminization of Soviet medicine has been related by many observers, including Navarro, to the specific value structure imposed on the labor force of Soviet society. Industrial production was given high priority, and hence "the second-rate workers—women—were to perform the second-rate jobs" (ibid.:48). Still Navarro interprets the figures on the female domination of the workforce of physicians as a sign of the emancipation of women. He suggests that "Soviet women have far more opportunities than women living in the capitalist world," a circumstance he extends to all socialist countries (ibid.:80).

The picture Navarro portrays of the work that Soviet women physicians do, however, bears a striking resemblance to the distribution of women in various medical specialties and practice settings that we are witnessing in today's medicine in most Western societies. Although the Soviet figures are high for that time, the trend is clearly visible: The higher the prestige of a field, the lower the proportion of women. For example, in the early 1970s, women constituted over 90 percent of the pediatricians, obstetricians-gynecologists, cardiorheumatologists, and endocrinologists, while they were only around 30 or 40 percent of the surgeons, who still enjoyed traditional high prestige (ibid.:78).

The unequal distribution of women health professionals in various practice settings and sectors of the health care system prevailed as well. As Navarro shows, women composed 85 percent of the health labor force in the Soviet Union in the early 1970s, but their proportion is lower the higher up one goes in the medical hierarchy. For example, in the mid-1970s, 10 percent of those in the Academy of Medical Services, 20 percent of the professors of medicine, 50 percent of the administrators, and 40 percent of tertiary-care physicians were women, as compared to 70 percent of the secondary-care physicians, 90 percent of the primary-care physicians, 85 percent of the feldshers, and 99.5 percent of the nurses (ibid.:76).

In a study conducted in 1991–1992 on men and women physicians practicing in the district of Moscow, the gender segregation of work of the 1970s portrayed above was confirmed (Kauppinen-Toropainen 1993; Kauppinen, Yasnaya, and Kandolin 1996). Men tended to practice in anesthesiology, surgery, psychiatry, and neurology, whereas women were found mainly in pediatrics, gynecology-obstetrics, and general practice. This same pattern of practice by specialty and gender was confirmed in a study of Estonian physicians conducted in 1991 (Barr 1995). The latter study also showed that women were more likely than men to practice in outpatient polyclinics and less likely than men to work in hospitals and special institutes.

In addition to differences in professional specialization, the study of Moscow physicians found that the material rewards for the work done varied by gender: Women's salaries were 65 percent of men's (Kauppinen et al. 1996:169). The most evident reason for this salary gap was the

*Table 5.2.* The Experience of Stress Symptoms Reported by Russian Physicians by Gender (Moscow Area, 1991–1992)

| | *Experience often or constantly (%)* | |
|---|---|---|
| *Type of psychological symptom* | *Women (n = 207)* | *Men (n = 110)* |
| Headaches | 30 | 12 |
| Sexual inadequacy | 30 | 5 |
| Lack of energy | 27 | 9 |
| Tiredness and exhaustion | 26 | 16 |
| High level of psychological stress | 42 | 35 |
| Severe decline of coping skills | 28 | 12 |

*Source:* Kauppinen et al. (1996:171).

marked difference in average weekly hours spent at work—the women worked thirty-six hours, the men worked forty-six. This difference reflects power difference between the two genders both at and off work. On the one hand, attractive jobs are those that require a strong commitment to work and provide high pay, jobs—such as top administration, research, academia—that the men tend to get. On the other hand, a traditional division of labor between men and women tends to prevail in Russia, where women are assigned the primary responsibility for the family household chores (Kauppinen-Toropainen 1993). A shorter work week is hence often "chosen" by professional women in order to juggle the demands of work and the family.

Despite the gender segregation of medical work and remuneration, the Moscow study documented that both men and women physicians were highly committed to their profession: 82 percent reported that they would not consider changing their profession (Kauppinen et al. 1996:169). Nevertheless, at the personal level, the gendered aspects of the work conditions seem to have taken their toll. Women physicians reported, on all psychological dimensions, a markedly lower quality of life than men physicians. For example, women two to three times as often as men reported that they often or constantly have headaches, experience sexual inadequacy, lack of energy, tiredness, stress, and reduced coping capacities (see Table 5.2).

## CONCLUSIONS

There are three features connecting the U.S. and Russian development in the nineteenth century: *populism, separatism,* and *foreign-based medical education.* First, both societies were characterized by populist sentiments in the early 1860s. In Russia, populism constituted the basis for an intellectual and youth movement, which emerged in the two chief cities, St. Petersburg and Moscow. The early populist movement in the United States was anti-intellectual and emerged in the countryside in the East and Midwest. Only during the later Progressive Era in the 1890s did social reform become part of the movement, which then also included the women's movement (Hofstadter 1955; Morantz-Sanchez 1985).

Second, women's entry into medicine lay firmly on the foundation of separatism as an organizing principle of society: there were men's and there were women's spheres. The United States and Russia can be said to share the condition of segregation and the segregated path that women in the early phases had to use in order to enter medicine. In Russia, women entered medicine by a dual route: State-supported separatist medical education and foreign-based coeducation in medicine. The state separatist policy acknowledged women's special skills and gender-segregated niche in society and formally educated them for this gender-specific task within the health care system. Women physicians were primarily educated to treat women's and children's health problems—a gender-segregated inclusion of women into medicine.

Third, the restricted and separatist character of medical education for women was also the reason for U.S. and Russian women's search for medical education abroad in high-standard coeducational medical faculties in Europe. Access to high-standard medical education abroad—notably in Switzerland and France—enabled women not only to receive basic medical education but, more importantly, to get clinical training.

Before the Russian revolution, the age of cottage industry medicine prevailed: Women were working as private physicians in the cities, mostly serving women and children. Some women ventured out as zemstvo physicians to the countryside, but it was mostly feldshers—a kind of physician assistant—who served the needs of the peasants and the country people. In fact, as historians have pointed out, a high proportion of the feldshers were women (e.g., Ramer 1990:123).

The common denominator of the Soviet and Scandinavian state-dominated medical mode of production was its decommodification: It became a service universally available to all citizens. But in contrast to Scandinavia, the state-dominated health care system in Soviet medicine came to change the character and gender of the medical profession in the Soviet Union fundamentally. In the Soviet Union, hospital medicine emerged with the industrialization of the rest of the society in the 1930s, but a perennial lack of resources never made this mode of production the nexus of scientific medicine as it was in Western societies. Instead, the medical profession was stripped of its privileged market and reduced to one employed group among other female-dominated health occupations in the public sector. During the era of Soviet medicine, medical societies and associations were outlawed, and a physician was but one of many occupations composing the state employees and medical workers. The medical profession did not control the training of its new members nor its own knowledge base. In 1988, in the whole Soviet Union, there were nine university-affiliated medical schools and eighty-four medical institutes (Barr 1995:375; Rayan 1989:4). Here the medical profession took the character that has been described as proletarianization and feminization.

In 1950, women constituted an overwhelming majority of the physicians in the Soviet Union. Yet, it was not the public sector per se—a central feature of Soviet medicine—and the physicians' status as state employees that transformed Russian medicine from a male-dominated to a female-dominated profession. Instead, it was two other social conditions of Soviet society that were conducive to this transition. First, after 1930, with the implementation of the New Economic Policy, industrial production was given a high priority, and so-called nonproductive activities like the service sector, including medicine, were given secondary importance in the hierarchy of values in the Soviet Union. Second, maternal and child health were high on the agenda in the postrevolutionary period. This women's health agenda had also been advanced by the pioneering women physicians in Russian medicine (Tuve 1984:116). But this agenda was gradually overshadowed by the emphasis in Soviet medicine on the industrial and hence male worker. By the 1930s, women physicians—although a majority of the medical practitioners—had lost their agenda and constituency to the goal of the industrialization of the Soviet Union. Lack of resources later resulted, however, in the demise of any—female or male—gender agenda in health.

As medicine had become a solidly female profession, gender still had a role in shaping the division of labor within medicine. Men have tended to work in prestigious specialties, in hospitals, and special institutes, while women have worked in primary care and in outpatient clinics, and been paid lower salaries.

The health care system stagnated severely during the Brezhnev period (from about 1964 to the early 1980s) when there was no investment nor development in medicine. Although the period of perestroika and glasnost infused a new vigor into Russian society, medicine was hardly affected. Instead, the percentage of the gross national product (GNP) going to health dropped: it was 6.6 percent in 1965, 4.5 percent in 1985, and declined to about 2 or 3 percent thereafter (Schultz and Rafferty 1990:194; Barr and Field 1996:308). Around 10 percent was spent on health care in most other Western societies.

During perestroika and glasnost, the overproduction of physicians and the past focus on the number of physicians as the symbol of the success of

Soviet medicine were reevaluated. Efforts to improve the quality of medical education and plans to reduce the enrollments of medical students were adopted by the Russian Health Ministry in 1992 (Rayan and Ray 1996:340).

When the Soviet Union collapsed, so did the foundation of its health care system. Since 1991, the route taken toward health insurance and a decentralized system have implied a public-private mixture of funding at the regional level, and the determination of the expenditures of these funds at the provincial level (Curtis, Petukhova, Sezonova, and Netsenko 1997; Burger, Field, and Twigg 1998; Twigg 2000). The right to private practice was instituted in 1993 by Article 56 of the so-called Law of Fundamentals of the Russian Federation's Legislation on the Protection of Citizens' Health, which also instituted a health care system based on universal, compulsory medical insurance. The insurance system is based on employers' paying a 3.6 percent payroll tax for their workers, with local governments' paying a per capita contribution for the nonemployed (Rayan and Ray 1996:342; Twigg 2000).

The decentralization of administration and financing and the emergence of insurance medicine has created a pluralistic system, a trend that has not yet meant an organization of medical practitioners as a strong professional body. The profession is characterized by internal fragmentation: it is divided into one hundred specialties.[2]

During the postcommunist era, the medical profession has remained a hybrid (Field 1991), i.e., it is powerful vis-á-vis patients but powerless as a collective and political body. Since the mid-1990s, the organization of physicians into a collective body for improving their work conditions, and their professional standing, and for asserting quality standards on their work has been further hampered by the perennial lack of funds for health care and regional variations in the remuneration of physicians. In this respect, the legal profession has been in a more advantageous position: Lawyers have benefited from the influx of foreign business and capital. The externally funded market has strengthened the lawyers' professional position (Schecter 2000:86). By contrast the financial crisis in 1997–1998 cut government financing by 18 percent, and hardest hit were health care workers, who have suffered from a lag in the payment of salaries (Twigg 2000:60–61).

Since the mid-1990s, a dual system has existed. Some physicians, as in the Moscow region, are still state employees and receive a salary for their work, other physicians are on payment schemes in group practices, and still others work in private practice (Barr and Field 1996:309; Burger et al. 1998:757). The private sector, of whom 40 percent are men, is small, comprising about 3 percent of the physicians (Luksha and Mansurov 1998). Although a majority of the medical practitioners are still women, the proportion of men has increased and men tend to occupy the prestigious positions. In 1960, 24 percent of doctors were men; in 1990, 31 percent were men (Table 5.1).

Yet the reforms in health care have so far focused merely on implementing new methods of health care financing rather than given similar attention to improving hygiene standards and to advancing ecological and public health programs (Twigg 1999:381). The latter endeavors would certainly improve the health of the Russians, whose health profile and life expectancy, especially that of men, have fallen dramatically over the past twenty years (Cockerham 1997, 1999; Chenet 2000; Field 2000). The figures on women's reproductive health are not very comforting either: since 1970 there have been more than twice as many officially registered abortions as there have been births (Field 2000:14). The use of contraceptives was rather limited still in 1994: 4 percent of women aged fifteen to forty-nine used oral contraceptives, and 20 percent used intrauterine devices (ibid.:14). As observers of Russian women's economic, political, and social position in postcommunist Russia have noted, poverty is hitting women particularly hard. It has been estimated that 90 percent of the unemployed in the cities are women. At the same time, child care centers have been closed en masse (five thousand in 1993 alone), thereby further marginalizing women on the labor market. In politics, women's representation in the Duma declined from 13 to 10 percent in 1995. The liberalization has generated a new tendency to objectify women, as is exemplified by an expanding market of pornography and sexual services, a trend that further weakens women's position in society (Sperling 2000).

## NOTES

1. The first cohort of women physicians to graduate from the women's medical course was an exception: as of 1882 more than half of the graduates first practiced in salaried positions as zemstvo physicians (Tuve 1984:769; Engel 1979:407).

2. As a comparison, Denmark had twenty-five specialties, Norway thirty, Finland forty-nine, and Sweden sixty-two in 2000 (Nordic Medical Associations 2000).

# 6

# Does Gender Matter?

## Women as Medical Practitioners

## INTRODUCTION

The gender segregation of medical work seems to be surprisingly common in most Western health care systems. As shown in the previous chapters, in the United States, Scandinavia, and Russia women physicians tend to work in general practice and specialties related to children, whereas surgery, especially, is male-dominated. This pattern prevails in other countries as well (Riska and Wegar 1993a)—for example, the United Kingdom, France, Australia (Pringle, 1998; Le Feuvre 1999; Crompton, Le Feuvre, and Birkelund 1999), Canada, and Belgium (De Koninck et al. 1997; Meeuwesen et al. 1991), and Japan (Long 1986). In health care systems with a tradition of entrepreneurial practice, men enter private practice more often than do women, while women tend to be overrepresented in salaried and part-time positions in more bureaucratic settings (Maheux, Dufort, Béland, Jacques, and Lévesque 1990; Kletke et al. 1996; McKinlay and Marceau 1998). As shown in Chapter 3, in the U.S. medical profession, the proportion of salaried physicians is much higher among women than men. In the Scandinavian countries where a majority of physicians are salaried and work in the public sector, women tend to be well represented in private practice. Furthermore, private practice is concentrated in urban areas and pursued by specialists.

Yet these studies on gender segregation of medical practice generally do not address the question of whether there are any differences in the way women and men practice within a special type of practice or medical specialty. Studies that have addressed this question are of two types: quantitative and qualitative. Besides representing different methodological approaches, they represent different theoretical traditions. Most of the quantitative studies take a nominal approach: they look at the sex composition of a specialty and map what kind of work women and men do. In the second category, studies have used qualitative methodologies in order to capture the cultural meanings embedded within existing rankings of specialties. Within the latter genre there are studies that examine the impact of gender on practice style. They suggest that the focus should not only be on the gender of the practitioner but also include an analysis of the embedded character of gender in the organization of medicine.

## QUANTITATIVE STUDIES: A NOMINAL APPROACH

"A nominal characteristic is any socially recognized attribute on which people are perceived to differ in a categorical rather than graduated or ordinal way" (Ridgeway 1991:368). The nominal approach implies that certain attributes, such as competence, become attached to nominal characteristics and are treated as separate from their embedded social context. Studies applying a nominal approach to the gender difference in medical practice began to be undertaken in the 1980s. Only studies done in the 1990s will be reported here, for a number of reasons. One reason is that since the 1990s a much higher proportion of physicians have been women. They can no longer be seen merely as tokens since they have a visible presence in most fields. Another reason is that most of the early studies were methodologically flawed, focusing merely on gender without controlling for practice setting, specialty, and type of patients. Conclusions were drawn about the impact of gender on medical practice when gender differences were found, although other confounding structural characteristics of medical practice were the more likely explanation for the documented gender differences.

Studies on gender and practice style done in the 1990s show four differences between men and women physicians: (1) style of communication with patients, (2) the functional division of labor, (3) the psychosocial effects of work, and (4) therapy decisions.

First, women tend to have better empathic skills in dealing with patients than do men. In their review of research on gender differences in patient-physician communication, Roter and Hall (1998) point to four major findings. First, female physicians use more partnership statements in their routine communication, thereby encouraging the patient to take a more active role. Second, female physicians are more likely to resort openly to textual or collegial knowledge in communicating with the patient. Third, female physicians tend, during a visit with the patient, to be less verbally dominant than male physicians. Fourth, female physicians do more probing of issues of a psychosocial nature and provide more psychosocial counseling.

For example, Canadian and Dutch studies have found that women physicians tend more than men to ask questions and provide information (Maheux et al. 1990; Meeuwesen, Schaap, and van der Staak 1991; Roter,

Lipkin, and Korsgaard 1991; Roter, Stewart, Putnam, Lipkin, Stiles, and Inui 1997; Bensing et al. 1993).

Women physicians' psychosocial and empathic skills have been confirmed in a number of studies. A Canadian survey study assessed patient care attitudes among family physicians in Ontario. Female physicians scored significantly higher on empathy than males, and women were also more likely than men to express strong interest in the psychosocial aspects of patient care (Williams 1999; for the United States, see West 1993). By contrast, an Israeli study on hospital physicians found no gender differences in compassionate-empathic behavior (Carmel and Glick 1996). The study measured the compassionate-empathic personality trait by means of a reputational method, i.e., as a colleague assessment, which was further verified by a self-assessment. This particular method might have influenced the measurement results for both genders.

In Canadian and Dutch studies across specialties, women physicians have been found to spend significantly more time with patients (Roter et al. 1991; Bensing et al. 1993; Meeuwesen et al. 1991; Roter and Hall 1998). Some scholars have attributed this finding to the fact that women physicians tend to see female patients, who generally have longer visits, and younger patients, who come for an initial visit. Women tend to provide more preventive services than do men, a feature that is also connected to their work with female and young patients (Bensing et al. 1993).

The selective character of patients tends to characterize particularly female-dominated practices and specialties. To account for the impact of the physician's gender, it is therefore important to examine studies in which a number of these factors have been controlled for. For example, a U.S. study on gender differences in practice style controlled for four conditions: gender of the physician and setting (primary care residents), gender of the patient, patient's health status, and inclusion of only initial patient visits (Bertakis et al. 1995). With the patient's health status controlled for, no gender differences in time spent with the patient were found among the primary-care residents. But the practice style differed—women physicians provided preventive services more than men did, gathered more family information, and got more information about the social milieu of the patient. Men physicians tended to focus on history taking. Patients were more satisfied with female physicians, and in fact history taking reduced patient satisfaction. The researchers concluded that practice style as such—focusing on family matters rather than taking the history of the patient—influenced patient satisfaction. This study included physicians who were in the same age cohort. Another study of U.S. and Canadian hospital- and community-based practices found that young female physicians were not particularly appreciated by patients, especially male patients (Hall et al. 1994).

Second, there seems to be a gender division of labor within specialties. A British study reported a marked segregation of tasks between female and male general practitioners. In practices where there were both men and women, the men tended to have primary responsibility for minor surgery, computers, administration, practice finance, staff employment, meeting with external visitors, and preparing the annual report. The women reported major responsibility only in the areas of personal problems of the staff, women's health, and prenatal work (Chambers and Campbell 1996: 293; for Canada, see also Williams 1999:112).

The marked division of labor by gender among general practitioners was also confirmed in an Australian study (Britt et al. 1996). It showed that women worked mainly with female health problems (genital, reproductive), and endocrine, psychosocial, and nutritional problems. Men focused on cardiovascular, musculoskeletal, male genital, skin, and respiratory problems. The researchers concluded that the increasing proportion of female general practitioners will further polarize problem management among general practitioners so that in the future there will be few competent general practitioners but instead they will be specialists by default (ibid.:414). This point is also made by Roter and Hall (1998:1096) in their review of the literature on gender and patient-physician communication. They suggest that female physicians will become de facto psychosocial experts in the care of patients since they will increasingly be given the primary responsibility for emotionally distressed patients as male physicians avoid these issues in their practice.

An interesting counterpoint is made by Elstad (1994) in his study of Norwegian women's preference for a male or female physician. Women's preferences on this issue were in a factor analysis found to be related to three profiles of the behavior of the physician: the caring, the democratic, and the traditional/dominant. Only those women who valorized the democratic physician profile preferred a woman physician. By contrast, the traditional profile was related to a preference for a male physician, while the caring physician—in the Norwegian context—was not associated with any gender. Elstad (ibid.:14) interprets the latter result as an indication of the male-gendered behavior of many women physicians: Norwegian women physicians are not particularly feminine—gender-stereotypically empathic or caring—in their professional behavior.

Third, the psychosocial conditions for work seem to be different for women and men physicians. A British study on male and female general practitioners found that women physicians derived more job satisfaction from working with patients than did men (Chambers and Campbell 1996). This finding was also documented in a U.S. study (McMurray et al. 2000) and in a Canadian study of family physicians (Williams 1999): Women physicians were more satisfied than men with their overall practice. The

Canadian study showed that men and women physicians were equally concerned about the changing status of the profession as a whole (ibid.:113).

A number of studies have documented higher levels of stress reported by women physicians than by men. In her study of U.S. physicians (in psychiatry, pediatrics, obstetrics-gynecology, and family practice), Gross (1992) found that time pressure was the stressor most frequently cited by men and by women (53 percent), with no substantial gender differences. The second most common area of stress was the doctor-patient relationship, which was far more often cited by men (51 percent) than by women (18 percent) (ibid.:109). By contrast, the responsibility inherent in the work of a physician and career/family conflict acted as stressors more for women than for men (36 versus 21 percent, and 44 versus 6 percent, respectively). Furthermore, men were three times as likely as women to be concerned with their inability to cure and with threats of malpractice. A later U.S. study of the psychosocial conditions of physicians has shown that women physicians experience lack of control over their work and more stress and burn-out symptoms than do men (McMurray et al. 2000).

In a review of Canadian, British, and U.S. research on gender differences in physician stress, Gross (1997) is perplexed by the discrepant findings. The explanation, she suggests, lies in the different methodological approaches: Those studies that documented gender differences used stress inventories or closed questions, while those studies that could not find any gender differences in physician stress used open-ended questions. Gross's conclusion is that the stress inventories and closed questions were based on work-related stressors typically reported by males and that these indicators resulted in underreporting by women due to the different kind of stressors that women encounter at work. For example, questions related to sexual harassment, family work load, lack of mentors, and adequate day care for preschool children are generally not included in stress inventories.

In contrast to most U.S. findings, recent studies of the psychosocial work environment of the Norwegian, Swedish, and Finnish physicians indicate that there are differences in physician stress by type of practice but not by gender (Arnetz 2001; Töyry et al. 2001). This finding would suggest three things that are not mutually exclusive. First, it could mean that women have early on made a career choice that enables them to combine family and work. Second, it could mean that women have been integrated in the work environment and are experiencing the same degrees of rewards and stressors as men. Third, it might mean that family policies (e.g., publicly supported day care, shorter work days for parents with preschool children, opportunities for legislated parental leave) to support working parents relieve particularly women from non-work-related stressors that impinge on their work.

The first argument is supported by the findings of a national survey of Finnish physicians' work conditions (Töyry et al. 2001). There were on average no major gender differences in the reported experience of stress or stressors—for example, in the extent that demands at work influenced family life and vice versa, satisfaction with work, experience of burn-out.

Women physicians were more likely than men, however, to report that they had adjusted their career to the demands of the family. For example, 17 percent of the women but 8 percent of the men had given up their job because their spouse's job required a move to another community. Similarly, 25 percent of the women but 6 percent of the men reported that they had worked part-time on account of family reasons.

Although on average there were no differences between Finnish women and men physicians' perception of a list of stressors—work, family matters, work matters, combining work and family matters, health, economic situation, other—there appeared interesting differences by age. Work was listed by both men (48 percent) and women (47 percent) as the factor causing most stress, but women aged 25–34 were more likely (53 percent) than men (43 percent) to report work as a major stressor. The situation was the reverse in the 55–65 age category (55 percent of the men versus 42 percent of the women). Family matters were seen by about 10 percent of men and women as the most important stressor, with a slight tendency for young men (10 percent) more often than young women (7 percent) to perceive this as a stressor, and for older women (15 percent) more often than older men (9 percent) to perceive family as a stressor. This result is quite different from the one that would have been expected from previous international research in the field. In response to the question on the capacity to juggle demands of work and family, a gender difference was found only for those in the age category 35–44 years, a group that could be expected to have small children: 52 percent of the women and 38 percent of the men reported that such conflicting demands caused most stress (Töyry et al. 2001). North-American studies have commonly reported a finding, especially, of gender differences in stress or work performance by marital status. U.S. and Canadian studies show that married women physicians must, much more than men, sacrifice their professional life, in terms of time at work and career ambitions, because of demands set by their role as spouse (Sobecks et al. 1999; Williams 1999; McMurray et al. 2000; Hinze 2000).

In this genre of studies on psychosocial work environment and stress a number of issues are still underresearched. An examination of the structural features of practice—for example, salaried status or entrepreneurial and group practice, or female-dominated, gender-balanced, or male-dominated practice—would yield interesting new information. Such structural features would provide information about the way the organization of and the normative features of work impinge on the expected performance of men and women physicians.

An issue that has had some media attention is the claim that women physicians have a higher suicide rate than men physicians. Lindeman et al. (1996), in their review of existing international research on this issue, found that this genre of research suffers from methodological problems. The small number of female cases in most countries and the lack of age-standardization of the numbers for men and women make any comparison between men and women physicians problematic. On the other hand, women physicians have been found to have a suicide rate significantly higher than that of other professional women.

Fourth, a number of studies have documented differences in the therapy decisions of men and women physicians. The overview presented here will focus on the two major areas of research that have sparked controversy and debate about the treatment of women's health needs: reproductive health matters and coronary heart disease.

## Reproductive Health Matters

A number of studies have shown than women physicians are more inclined than men physicians to provide preventive services to women. For example, American women were found to be more likely to undergo screening with Pap smears and mammograms if they saw female rather than male physicians (Lurie et al. 1993). It has been suggested that findings like these are related to the perception of women who come for a gynecological examination and who consider female physicians more attentive and informative than men (van Elderen, Maes, Rouneau, and Seegers 1998). A U.S. study explored this finding further in order to examine whether gender differences in screening were related to different types of patient populations seen by men and women physicians. The provision of mammography was found not to be related to demographic or attitudinal differences between their patient populations (Andersen and Urban 1997).

A Finnish study found more similarities than differences between male and female physicians regarding menopausal and postmenopausal hormone therapy, and obstetrical and contraceptive practices. The study reviewed five Finnish surveys conducted in 1988 and 1989: the groups included were medical students, gynecologists, internists, obstetricians, and general practitioners. The overall findings were that women physicians and women medical students were more likely to recommend prescribing of hormones, the women obstetricians were twice as likely as men obstetricians to suggest that labor be induced for convenience of the patients, and women physicians were inclined to offer more alternatives for contraception than men physicians (Mattila-Lindy et al. 1997).

The foregoing studies were based on attitudes and therapy decisions in hypothetical patient cases. Dulmen and Bensing (2000) compared videotapes of real-life outpatient encounters ($N = 303$) with female and male

gynecologists in the Netherlands. Their results showed that female gynecologists did longer physical examinations, asked fewer questions, had
longer conversations with their patients, and communicated both verbally
and nonverbally in a more affective way. Male gynecologists asked more
medical questions and gave more medical advice. In a multilevel regres-
sion analysis, however, the gender difference in affective communication
behavior disappeared. Dulmen and Bensing found the tendency for
female gynecologists to ask fewer medical questions to be related to the
patient's greater willingness to provide information for which the male
physician had to probe. As other studies—primarily U.S., Canadian, and
Dutch—have shown, the encounter with female physicians is characterized by a more empathic and active listening than with male physicians
(e.g., West 1993; Roter and Hall 1998; Dulmen and Bensing 2000).

Nevertheless, it is important to recognize that the provision of preventive services and information is not merely related to the gender of the
physician but to the structure of the health care system as well. Zimmerman and Hill (2000:779) make the observation that changes in the provision of health care to American women over the past two decades relate to
structural changes in U.S. health care: women are receiving more preventive care as a result of managed-care plans.

## Coronary Heart Disease

The different kind of treatment for men and women who suffer from
coronary heart disease has been another major area of research that has
illustrated women's unmet health needs.

Despite the decreasing cardiovascular disease mortality in most Western
societies, the leading cause of death, at least in the United States, is still cardiovascular disease, regardless of gender. In 1997, cardiovascular disease
accounted for 43 percent of all deaths in women in the United States (Nabel
2000:572). The alert to this trend in the late 1980s set in motion a movement
to include women and members of minority groups in clinical research
funded by the National Institutes of Health, a policy that was enacted in
1990 in the United States (see also Chapter 8). This program seems to have
been successful: women were enrolled in trials at rates that exceeded the
prevalence of cardiovascular disease among women in the general population during 1965 and 1998 (Buring 2000).[1] A number of large follow-up
studies are currently ongoing to test for major risk factors and the prevalence of heart disease among American women. The fourteen-year follow-
up on lifestyle-related risk factors—smoking, overweight, lack of exercise,
and poor diet—in the so-called Nurses' Health Study in the United States
showed that women who had none of the measured lifestyle risk factors
had a 83 percent lower risk of coronary events than the rest of the women

(Nabel 2000). It is therefore important that physicians alert women, not only men, to the importance of preventive measures.

A number of studies have provided extensive reviews on the gender differences in preventive, acute, and rehabilitative measures for men and women suffering from coronary artery disease (Haas 1998; Lorber 2000a; Dulmen and Bensing 2000; Zimmerman and Hill 2000). These reviews suggest that women tend to receive fewer services and interventions than men. Some studies have suggested that men physicians tend to be inattentive to women's symptoms and health needs related to heart disease (e.g., McKinlay 1996).

In order to provide evidence of gender bias in the diagnosis and management of patients, Case, Hatala, Blake, and Golden (1999) examined the responses of U.S. and Canadian medical students ($N = 3,059$, of whom 41 percent were women) to twenty-seven patient-vignette cases, in which the gender of the patient randomly was shown as male or female. The overall finding was that women and men students were more likely to answer correctly if the case was a male patient than if the case was a female patient. Three cases portrayed patients with heart problems. In the case of the patient having congestive heart failure, women students were more alert than the male students in diagnosing this problem correctly both in the female and male case. In the two other cases, the heart problem of the male and female case was combined with another health problem. In these cases, no significant differences in the correct diagnosis appeared between men and women students.

## QUALITATIVE STUDIES: THE EMBEDDED APPROACH

The nominal approach to gender and practice style tend to make invisible the underlying gendered character of medicine and the gendered character embedded in specialties. The embedded approach to gender in medicine implies that gender is viewed as built into the operation of medicine and is part of a tacit understanding of how medicine as an institution is organized. The tacit character of gender implies that certain values and procedures are seen as normal and totally gender-neutral ways of organizing activities.

The term *gendered* here means a set of values about the ranking of gender. Such a ranking creates a structure of gender relations, a structure built on gender inequality (Acker 1992; Lorber 1994:14). The strength of this perspective is that it redirects the focus of the analysis from individual traits and choices in medicine to the gendered processes and gendered practices of power built into medicine as an organization. The embedded approach enables researchers to explain how two social institutions—the gender system and medicine—are interrelated. The weakness of this approach is that it contains an a priori hypothesis that tends to be confirmed. But the purpose of this kind of research, as Britton (2000:430) reminds us, is not to find the ultimate, "ungendered" form of organization but rather to try to identify "less oppressively gendered forms" of organizations.

In the 1980s, a number of qualitative studies examined the cultural meanings embedded in medical practice. In focus was the "culture of medicine" and the way that medical experts defined their expertise not only among themselves but also vis-à-vis their clients. This genre of research documented the element of professional dominance involved in the construction of the medical knowledge of and boundaries of medical experts vis-à-vis other health professionals (e.g., Silverman 1987; Mishler 1984). In the 1990s, the symbolic interactionist approach of earlier studies was superseded by a phenomenological approach that focused on the social-discursive organization of medicine. A social-constructionist or an explicitly Foucauldian analysis of medical discourse became the theoretical framework for the examination of medicine as a cultural system. The studies documented how certain social practices created a cultural unity among experts in a subdiscipline of medicine. Here the liturgy of these practices was mapped: the ritualized performances and talk of the specialists in a field of medicine (e.g., Atkinson 1995; Fox 1992).

A number of these studies, like many feminist studies in the past, assumed that the gender dimension rested in the interaction between the male-physician and the female-patient. In these studies, relations among physicians were portrayed as gender-neutral rather than another gendered cultural element inscribed in medicine. Furthermore, gender is not only a question of the masculine and feminine character of practice but a structure that forms the social and technical division of labor within medicine.

The embedded approach to gender is represented in two different inquiries regarding the structure and operation of medicine: some studies have examined how specialties are gendered, and others have tried to identify the gender discourses about medical practice. Recent qualitative studies on women physicians' practice in male- or female-dominated practices have suggested that the specialties themselves are gendered and that a masculine ethos or values are embedded in the way that medicine is practiced in most specialties. While the early studies tended to see women physicians as victims of a massive male enterprise of medicine, more recent studies have tended to give women voices as they encounter in their daily practice the male-gendered master status of their profession and their male colleagues' and clients' reactions to their female gender. Women physicians are portrayed as actively constructing their own meanings and their own definitions of the situation. This kind of approach has examined two polar types of practices: either highly male-dominated specialties like surgery, or specialties where women are very well represented like general practice.

## The Masculine Ethos of Surgery

Surgery has recently been the focus of a number of studies, because of surgery's particular medical culture (Fox 1992; Pringle 1998; Conley 1998; Katz 1999; Cassell 2000). One of these reports differs, though, from the standard research format on account of its cause célèbre: Frances K. Conley entered Stanford University School of Medicine in 1961, where she continued her career on the faculty from 1975 until she resigned in May 1991 from her position as a tenured full professor of neurosurgery. Her reminiscences about her career in medicine (Conley 1998) constitute a true tale of the conditions under which women pursued a career in U.S. medicine in the 1970s and 1980s. She describes how she as a token woman felt entering into medicine and "growing up" to be a neurosurgeon—how she became "one of the boys." According to her, women and men were early channeled into different paths in medicine, but this selective recruitment was never articulated even though a separation based on gender was openly practiced. Women medical students learned early that only a few specialties were open to them—pediatrics, psychiatry, general internal medicine, family practice. Unconsciously Conley accommodated her professional life to the prevailing macho culture. This culture normalized the display of male sexuality as part of the interaction with any woman in the medical school and hospital setting. Touching of women students' and nurses' bodies and sexual innuendo were presented by the male physicians as the normal working of the university hospital or medical school, even though these actions were blunt examples of the micropolitics of male power.

Conley's initial negative reactions to the power exerted by the medical men were mollified by the intense social pressure of adjustment to the general pace of medical school education, which she describes as a demoralizing, dehumanizing process that left no time for emotion for humanity—neither for men nor women. As a token woman, her survival strategy was the one of "blending in": "Through subtle unconscious social pressure, it seemed more important to be regarded as 'one of the boys' than to be seen running around with a bunch of women" (Conley 1998:28). It is obvious from her text that—although she did not understand it at the time—the "boys" did not see her as one of them (Cassell 2000:210). Conley identified herself as marginal by the mere fact that she was a pioneer in her field. Even later, when she recognized the gendered character of her work environment, Conley did not protest because she took for granted that as women were increasing in the profession, they would advance to all ranks. In this way, the problems that she as a female pioneer in neurosurgery had experienced would automatically wither away. (This is the theory of the representational lag of women in medicine and the sociology of numbers argument presented in Chapter 2.) Yet Conley's own career reached the point where she realized that what she had perceived as her private problem of being a pioneer in her field was not at all a private problem of an individual woman. Instead, it was a public issue of sexual harassment that women have to endure in the male-gendered organization of medicine.

But Conley's tale is also one that brings the reader's attention to the importance of male mentors. Her career is at all times dependent on male mentors. In fact, her career gets a problematic twist when one of her mentors turns against her. This circumstance is also evident in the historical accounts of the careers of individual women in medicine (e.g., Drachman 1984; More 1999) and also in later reportings in the genre of women physicians' narratives. For example, Cassell's (2000) description of one woman surgeon's career in a southern medical school—presented as "a worst-case scenario"—is almost a replica of Conley's story of how a former male mentor turns against his female protégé because the male mentor suddenly perceives the female research partner as a serious academic competitor rather than as the subservient collaborator she once was.

Cassell's (2000) book *The Woman in the Surgeon's Body* is an interesting reading parallel to the gender-neutral analysis of surgery provided by Fox (1992), reported in *The Social Meaning of Surgery*, and Katz's (1999) work *The Scalpel's Edge: The Culture of Surgeons*. The focus of these studies is the unique culture of surgery and how surgical authority is constituted. Cassell, Fox, and Katz have all adopted a social-constructionist view. Although both Fox and Katz are explicitly interested in the cultural aspects of the so-called surgical personality, they leave its gendered aspects unexamined. Cassell, Fox, and Katz report on the rituals and rhetorical markers of the "circuit of hygiene" (Fox 1992:15) and its gendered elements (e.g., the ritual of the scrub, separate changing rooms and dress for men and women, whereby women surgeons become equated with nurses). While Fox and Katz portray these activities as a way of inscribing into discourse a particular set of social relations between patients, surgeons, and other staff, Cassell perceives the same activities as a way of not only "doing surgery" but, more importantly, of "doing gender."

But Cassell—likewise Hinze (1999) in her study of resident physicians, most of whom were in surgery residencies—does not describe gender as a mere performance but also as an embodied status. The physical appearance of being a male and a surgeon constitutes the master status of surgery. Both Cassell and Hinze conclude that the skills and knowledge valorized in surgery are embodied: The "good hands" of the surgeon are those of a man. But they also suggest that the kind of authority and professional prestige enjoyed by surgeons rests on values and symbolism that are culturally masculine: A surgeon is connected with a masculine ethos of hardness, calculation, and instrumentality (Katz identifies the masculine ethos but does not pursue gender further in the analysis of her findings). The masculine ethos is captured in two social types of surgeon whom Cassell calls the "iron surgeon" and "the Hemingwayesque surgeon" to indicate the authoritarian character of the former and the potent and egocentric macho personality of the latter.

But as both Cassell (2000:67–76) and Pringle (1998:91) show in their studies of women surgeons, women are channeled into certain gendered niches, like breast surgery. In breast surgery, being a woman is considered an advantage. Yet for many women, as for men, breast surgery was not their first choice. It is considered a technically boring and routine operation and hence of low prestige in the ranking of surgical procedures. As Cassell shows, the symbolic and cultural significance of the breast for the patient creates a difficult situation for the men (or any surgeon, regardless of gender), for whom this body part is "just" a breast (see also Katz 1999:10).

The Scandinavian studies that have examined women physicians' status in surgery confirm the foregoing portrayal of surgery in the U.S. studies. There was pressure to conform to the master status of the surgeon—a physically strong man who could handle the hard work of surgery. As one of the women surgeons in Nore's (1993:35) Norwegian study remembers:

> I was thin as a piece of paper when I graduated. I lifted weights for ten years to be strong enough for surgery. . . . It was quite funny, but then I began to get muscles in my back. It was long before they'd invented this body building! I was ashamed and stopped. But I'd become strong enough and it wasn't so bad.

The physical proficiency and the cultural attributes of the male surgeons were for women surgeons a muster to pass, but even Cassell concludes that the women surgeons were on average different. Her finding was that the women related in a caring, compassionate way to their patients and did not merely view them as bodies (Cassell 2000:130). In the Scandinavian studies on this topic, women surgeons have also argued that they as women have different values and relate to medicine and patients differently than men. A Swedish female orthopedist reflects on her choice of specialty:

> I think I chose orthopedics not because I thought it was so incredibly important to be a big surgeon. I don't believe that and that it's so important to do operations—I don't think so. I'm not that hot on using the scalpel, as some people are.

I think that I'm trying to introduce a little humanism into orthopedics also, and I think it's fun because it's such a positive specialty. One can do a lot for the patients. (Einarsdottir 1997:258)

The women surgeons examined in Nore's study in Norway had similar views:

It depends to what extent a female surgeon maintains that we [women] have to establish norms that are different . . . in addition to the professional [characteristics]. It's like women clergy—the education is the same and the task is the same and many say that the women clergy say it in a different way and they do it in a different way because they constitute a different section of the population. . . . I feel that women can contribute something [special to surgery]. (1993:42)

A Finnish woman physician in general practice considered women physicians in general to be driven by other motivations in their work, which made them underrepresented in fields like surgery. As she reflected:

Something that I also believe has an impact is that women don't experience a similar pressure to practice heroic medicine like surgery. The reason why women don't chose a career in surgery I believe has to do with the fact that that they don't have such a need to be recognized or to hold the healer's knife in their hand. In some way men have different reasons for studying medicine. I believe they are more success-oriented and have a clear sense of what a successful physician is like. (Riska and Wegar 1995:207)

## The Holistic and Female Approach to Medicine: Women General Practitioners

In addition to studies on the male-dominated and male-gendered specialty of surgery, the embedded approach to medical practice is represented by studies that have examined specialties in which women are well represented, like general practice.

In her study of women general practitioners in Britain, Brooks (1998) distinguished between two major types of strategies among women general practitioners to deal with gender in the division of labor in medical work. One strategy of the women physicians was to embrace a view on their practice that negated any influence of gender on their work. This attitude—the general GP—embraced a generalist role resembling the traditional family GP. These women physicians argued that they "happened" to be women. They did not think that gender restricted or guided their practice of medicine. Another strategy—the women's GP—was adopted among women physicians accepting the feminized element of the work and willing to do emotional work and women's health. The women's GPs were further divided into two groups: The committed women's GP and the natural women's

*GP*. The committed women's GP was characterized by a feminist and political commitment to women's health issues. The natural women's GPs based their views about their professional role on a belief in a "natural" gender division of labor. The women who held this essentialist notion of gender assumed that women by virtue of their special female skills and values were more suited than men to undertake certain tasks (see also the cultural feminist and managerial-diversity theories on this issue in Chapter 2).

In her interview study of British and French women physicians, Le Feuvre (1999) used the concept "gender ethos" to describe the degree to which women physicians conform to or contest the legitimacy of the binary gender division. She distinguishes three types of gender ethos: the constructivist, the normative, and the transgressional. The *constructivist gender ethos* resembles Brooks' generalist GP category: These women resisted the gender differentiation process and suggested that physician's work is a gender-neutral skill and a physician is always first a physician and secondly a woman. As for gender of the physician, it was assumed that men and women were interchangeable. The *normative gender ethos* accepted the feminine qualities of the work and saw female gender as an additional strength of medical practice. These women prioritized their family life above their professional life. Their view of gender was that there were real gender differences, and this view on difference influenced their choice of specialty and the way they practiced medicine. The *transgressional gender ethos* embraced the binary notion of gender—men and women as different—but women physicians holding this view were critical of the segregating effects of the gender process. Le Feuvre (ibid.:211) concludes that the normative gender ethos was far more prevalent in France than in Britain. It is suggested that this finding is related to the different organization of specialists in the two countries. Le Feuvre points out that specialists work in private practice in France and therefore have more autonomy to adjust their work schedule and work conditions than do specialists in the male-mainstream career pattern expected of specialists in the public sector in Britain.

## CONCLUSIONS

The studies on gender and practice style reviewed in the first section of this chapter have been quantitative. Much of this research has adopted a nominal approach to gender. A focus on the sex composition of specialties has a tendency to create a dichotomy between men's and women's practice styles and to homogenize women physicians. This approach easily leads to two conclusions about the impact of gender. First, if any gender differences are found, they are proof that gender matters; and, second, if no gender differences are found, this is evidence that gender does not matter or that gender equality has been achieved (e.g., Williams 1999:108; Kimmel 2000:512).

Although the results generally are descriptive, there is a certain tacit explanation of women's physicians' behavior or attitudes: gender socialization has formed women's and men's attitudes and choices. Hence, socialization theory and sex-role theory tend to serve as the tacit theoretical framework for this genre of studies.

The typologies constructed by Cassell, Brooks, and Le Feuvre represent the embedded approach to medical specialties and medical practice. According to this approach, medicine is perceived as imbued with masculine values and the practice of medicine captures these values. As women have entered medicine, these values have come to be associated with the ranking of specialties. Some specialties, like surgery, are perceived as capturing the masculine and embodied character of medicine. For Cassell (2000), a woman surgeon is never a gender-neutral surgeon, but her primary status will always be graded on her gender as that of a woman.

The foregoing studies all point to the masculine images and symbols that are embedded in most medical specialties and act as a cultural barrier with which women physicians early in their career are confronted. The studies do not, however, portray women as mere victims of the sex-typing of specialties and as passive objects of the gender system and larger health care system and the social differentiation taking place within these systems. Instead they suggest that women physicians construct their own discourses and strategies whereby they actively resist and reject the masculine culture of medicine. According to this approach, women physicians are both subjects and objects of social practices that shape their work conditions, professional interactions, and professional identity. Furthermore, women physicians are not treated as a homogeneous group sharing a common and universal female culture. Instead of one "female voice of medicine," the studies are suggesting that women physicians speak with the voices of many different kinds of women.

The next chapter will illuminate how gendered social practices shape the work of women working as pathologists. I will show that masculinity is still embedded in pathology but that this feature is quite successfully resisted by the women practitioners in this specialty.


## NOTE

1.   Although women are taking part in clinical trials funded by NIH grants, most reports are not adopting an analysis of the data by gender. A study of NIH-funded, non-sex-specific studies published in major U.S. medical journals (*New England Journal of Medicine, Journal of the American Medical Association, Journal of the National Cancer Institute, Circulation*) between 1993 and 1998 showed that even though 80 percent of the articles included women, only 25 to 30 percent of the studies with women subjects reported a gender analysis, e.g., a statement that there were no significant gender differences (Helmuth 2000:1562).

# 7

# New Pioneers: Women in Pathology

## INTRODUCTION

The preceding chapters have examined women physicians' careers in medicine from a macrolevel perspective. This chapter addresses the same issues from a microlevel perspective.

Here the concept of work and its gendered character is approached by means of the medical culture of pathology. Work in pathology has been associated with a certain master status and related masculine traits (Hughes 1958): A pathologist is a medical man who does autopsies and whose gender traits of fearlessness and emotional detachment from the tasks he is doing define the characteristics needed for the work (Hafferty 1988). Pathology has in a sense been delegated the "dirty work" of medicine (see Hughes 1958:52). Nonetheless, pathology has always had a certain aura of prestige since its practitioners have been assigned the task of providing the final diagnosis: the ultimate scientific truth of the etiology of a fatal case. There is, however, a clear division of labor between the experts on fatal diagnoses: Those who have specialized in pathology and those who work in forensic medicine. The former provide the etiology for a normal or natural death, whereas the latter are involved in examining those deaths assumed to be associated with a crime or not caused by a "natural" etiology. The study reported in this chapter covered pathologists only, i.e., those who provide the etiology of diseases causing a "natural" death or fatal diagnosis.

But pathology as a field has changed dramatically over the past decades. The changes in medicine and the refocusing on the biomedical aspects of medicine as the strength of the medical profession have moved the "dirty work" of pathology into the forefront of medical research. Today pathology mostly involves work at the microscope and the clerical work of writing reports on the character of tissue samples taken from live patients who have had or are undergoing surgery or screening. Today the task of the pathologists is, however, increasingly not to determine pathological tissues but to confirm the normality of the tissues of living patients. In this regard, work has changed from routinization of fatal diagnoses to confirming normality.

The unique feature of pathology is that the work does not involve any social interaction with patients or with colleagues representing other specialties. Work is done alone or, in diagnosing ambiguous tissue samples, as teamwork with other pathologists. In this sense, pathology, in the division of medical labor, is a domain structurally isolated from clinical work. Pathology is attached by outsiders to certain emotions—fears and myths—related to closeness to death and dying: about corpses, tumors, cancer, miscarriages, rejected implants. The structural separation and the symbolic content of pathology are two traits conducive to the emergence of shared experiences among those working in the field.

In contrast to most of the early work in the sociology of professions (e.g., Parsons 1951), Hughes (1958) brought attention to the importance of gender in the definition of the central characteristics of an occupational group (see Chapter 2). The "master status" of a profession captures the central traits associated with its incumbents, and male attributes have generally been viewed as congruent with the traits of the traditional professions. For those whose gender or race is deviant, the resulting status inconsistencies can pose a dilemma in doing the work. More recently the term "doing gender" (West and Zimmerman 1987) has been used to capture the processual aspect of gender: gender is constructed in social interaction rather than viewed as a static trait. The social construction of the gendered traits of special groups of physicians—for example, general practitioners (West 1993; Brooks 1998; see also Pringle 1998) and surgeons (Cassell 2000)—have been in focus in some recent studies as shown in Chapter 6. However, gender is still an issue underresearched in the sociological work on medical specialties. Consequently, feminist researchers (West 1993:64; Hinze 1999) have called for systematic research on how prevailing normative conceptions of gender form the work in different medical specialties.

Considering the values of emotional detachment associated with the field of pathology, it is not surprising to find that the field is not a top choice of medical students selecting a residency. Women physicians are generally found in medical specialties—like pediatrics, psychiatry, general practice, and geriatrics—that arguably fit their assumed empathic and interactive skills (see Chapter 6). It is for this reason that women who have specialized in pathology are pioneers: they are breaking gender-stereotypical notions about the master status of the pathologist, and they are also doing work viewed as providing new responses to many life-threatening diseases. Nevertheless, the proportion of women in pathology seems to vary widely from country to country. For example, women constitute about one-fourth of the specialists in pathology in the United Kingdom (Pringle 1998:104–5); 28 percent in Finland, Norway, Sweden, and the United States; and as high as 41 percent in Denmark (see Tables 3.4 and

4.2). The figures are changing rapidly in U.S. medicine: In 1998, 45 percent of the residents in pathology were women (AMWA 2000:2).

Although "nature" in the form of the biological raw material of the human body constitutes the allegedly gender-neutral domain assigned to the work of the pathologists, a social organization of work and an internal differentiation have emerged that are inscribed by a gendered culture. As the following sections will show, gender is embedded in how work in pathology is constructed, and gendered discourses are central for how work is defined and constructed for and by women pathologists. There are certain narrative and rhetorical devices whereby women pathologists legitimate and construct gender and work in pathology.

## THE SETTING AND METHODS

Why then do women venture into pathology, which is still heavily associated with masculine values and stereotypic notions about the manly qualities needed for doing the work? The issue can be illuminated by the accounts of some informants among women pathologists practicing in Finland. The health care setting in Finland was selected for two reasons. As shown in Chapter 4, in 2000, already half of the members of the medical profession in Finland were women. Still only 28 percent of the pathologists were women, which is one of the lowest percentages, outside surgery (14 percent), among existing medical specialties. In most primary-care specialties, women account for about 60 to 85 percent of the physicians.

At the time of this study in 1998, forty-one women worked in pathology in Finland. For the purpose of this study, ten women were initially selected from the list of pathologists appearing in the official catalog of *Physicians 1997–1998* issued by the Department of Health and Welfare in Finland. This catalog lists physicians by specialty, by last name in alphabetical order, and by rank and place of work. The women selected for interviews were chosen to represent different age groups, work settings, ranks, and regions of the country. The interviews were conducted from November 1998 to the beginning of February 1999. One of the women had moved abroad, and so another woman in a similar position was selected; and one woman did not want to be interviewed. Hence, this study is based on interviews with nine informants. This group proved to be sufficiently large, and in the last two interviews a certain saturation was apparent as the same themes that had emerged in the preceding interviews were repeated, and no substantially new information appeared. Each interview was conducted at a time and place convenient for the informant. The interviews lasted on average forty minutes.

Semistructured, the interviews followed a list of thirteen questions that covered seven main themes: the motives for selecting pathology as a specialization, the existence of gendered tracks during specialization, the organization of work and internal differentiation in pathology, work culture and language, the existence of men's and women's work in pathology, the reasons for the small number of women in the field, and future challenges of the field. The interviews were transcribed verbatim. The main themes were analyzed and coded, using an inductive approach (Glaser and Strauss 1967). The numbers indicated in the text after the citation from the informants' account are used throughout the chapter to refer to the informant in question.

## ATTRACTION TO THE FIELD: VISUALIZATION OF DISEASE

The field of pathology does not constitute a main draw for women entering medicine but is a field that later emerges as a choice of specialization. As one woman said, "Many know that they want to become pediatricians almost before they are born [laughs]—nobody for sure begins to study medicine because she wants to become a pathologist" (#1). Almost without exception the informants themselves brought up the regular hours of the work and the lack of on-call duty at night as one of the reasons for getting into the field. This reason was important for those who wanted to establish a family and have children. A certain sense of autonomy and control over the professional demands of work were stated as the reason for choosing pathology as a specialization. The lack of autonomy and control has been noted as a universal trend in current medical work, a trend that has been described as a social transformation or loss of the golden age of doctoring (see Chapter 2; see also McKinlay and Stoeckle 1988; McKinlay and Marceau 1998).

But equally important was the fact that pathology represented a particular approach to medicine: visualization of disease. Clinical work implied a large patient load in a health center setting, quick decisions, and no possibility of exploring the science aspects of illnesses. In contrast, pathology provided an opportunity to explore details and to be concerned with the specifics of diseases in which the informants were interested. The decontextualized body, represented by a tissue sample under the microscope, was the locus of information about disease. Through a reading of the tissues, the pathologist could see the body in a new way. In fact, the tissue was a representation of the body and through a reading of the tissue the body was made legible. In this way, both the normal and the pathological could be discerned.

Certain aesthetic values were related to this kind of diagnostic work focusing on details: There was a visual aspect and attraction in microscopy:

In fact, what originally interested me in pathology was that it is so visual. I could see this kind of electromicroscopy pictures of kidneys, and to me it was very exciting and beautiful. (#7)

Already when I was studying I realized that I saw things in the microscope much better than my fellow students. So in this respect I clearly had a kind of visual memory, and this is visual work. Another thing, certainly, was that when I saw patients at the health center, I always had the sense that I did not know [the diagnosis] for sure, but if I could open up and see, then I would know what there was. (#9)

The informants considered that the clinical gaze involved with patient work is too complex and uncertain to master because the sick person as a whole, including external social aspects, has to be considered. In order to read the body and to reach an "accurate" diagnosis, a visual exploration of the interior of the body is needed.

The "microscopic gaze" (Atkinson 1995) enables the pathologist to explore the body through the lens of the microscope. This is a view characterized as medical reductionism, suggesting that the etiology of disease can be reduced to a single cause and that that cause is inherent in the body. For the informants, the truth about disease was to be found in the uninhabited body—the corpse, the organs, the tissues. This required an interest in the observations of the details of even fragments of organs and tissues:

It always bothered me in patient work that treatment is based to a large extent on a certain notion that symptoms have usually been taken care of in a certain way and the diagnosis has been this or that. What attracts me in pathology is that I really see the organ and tissue changes. I'm perhaps a kind of theoretical type. My attention is drawn to details. (#1)

The work is rather independent and one can to some extent influence how work is done. . . . It suits me that it's this kind of precision work concerned with small details. And then that you can take your time and ponder the problem and not have to make a decision in a horrible hurry, as you have to in clinical work, where you have to make a quick decision whether the patient needs treatment. (#4)

After I graduated, I planned a patient-oriented specialty and I worked for some time in internal medicine at a large hospital. In fact, I'm sure that this was the time when I decided to become a pathologist. . . . In internal medicine I somehow experienced that there was too much of something other than medicine there. . . . I was perhaps . . . I was very young then and I felt I was not perhaps mature enough for it and these people had all kinds of problems that were not by any means medical problems and then—and then also you had to decide about all kinds of social benefits and write various kinds of certificates. I was more interested in the issue [scientific medicine] itself. (#7)

For the informants, the body's tissues are inscribed by disease, and only by a visual exploration of the tissues is the reading of the truth about the disease accomplished. In this process, the informants perceived themselves as passive readers of the truth as inscribed in the tissues. But as readers of the "principle of tissual communication" (Foucault 1975:149), pathologists are applying the discourse of pathology to construct bodies that are, however, representations of bodies from medical texts. Their craft is a visual skill composed of a shared language about the character of the tissues as matter and as objects. Pathologists have learned and continue to construct in their work a shared language about the normal and the pathological that they are visualizing. This information has to be conveyed to the clinician. Their own written case reports to the clinicians further reconstruct and confirm the body as a representation and as a text.

## THE MASTER STATUS: THE GENDERED CHARACTER OF AUTOPSIES AND MICROSCOPY

To outsiders, women's work in pathology seemed to be the antithesis of what woman physicians were supposed to do: women's skills are envisioned as holistic and caring rather than reductionistic and instrumental. Pathology is a field in which interactive skills for dealing with patients are not needed. Hence, women entering this field were often asked to give a rationale for why they had ventured into a field heavily associated with masculine values and attributes. The social reaction to their decision to specialize in pathology was one of amazement:

> I do remember that I was [laughs] leaving the health center to go to try [pathology] out. When I said "work in the pathology unit," everybody was totally horrified. The women said, "No, no it can't be true, you can't do that, that's awful." But I don't understand why only women would be afraid—or I don't know whether it's a matter of being afraid. On the other hand, it might be that women typically are such social beings, they have such social skills for interacting with patients that they do well on the clinical side [laughs]. They don't have the need to come to the pathology unit to work. Here we don't interact with the patients. (#6)

> Doctors—certainly a large proportion of them—have a need to do caring and verbal work. So pathology is this kind of specialty that fits research types who don't want to be treating patients. (#9)

The status incongruence of being a woman and being a pathologist was noted by the informants:

Well . . . sometimes [men] are very surprised: "Oh, you're a doctor" . . . "Oh, you're a pathologist" . . . they're surprised. That's their first reaction. (#5)

The social reaction that the women pathologists had encountered was a certain representation of pathology, an outdated male-constructed version of the work as doing autopsies. While this was still in many ways the master status of the specialty, this "dirty work" in fact defined the core of the professional skills of the pathologists. Doing autopsies was the arena where the diagnostic skills and the craftsmanship of the trade were originally learned. Doing autopsies was part of the early socialization of the visual skills in pathology—a shared collective recognition of the normal and pathological character of organs and tissues. This kind of visual skill was confirmed when the pathologist did this as routine work by him- or herself. The women pathologist themselves did not consider autopsy assignments low-status work but instead an essential part of maintaining the professional competence of a pathologist.

Yet, most women pathologists were caught by the outdated lay notion—one held among physicians and medical students as well—of the pathologist's work:

I think it's . . . that . . . during their early education the future physicians had taken in a very autopsy-focused image, and the same image that laypeople have: This kind of nut down in the basement who works alone with the dead—well, it's somehow stayed in the unconscious. (#2)

I'm sure that among laypeople and even among an incredibly large proportion of physicians, there's this notion that it's somehow macabre and sick and bewildering. They don't come to think of this microscope side at all but first only of the autopsy—that it's awful, "I *can't* do it, *how* can you do it?" [laughs]. (#1)

Yet, this masculine image of working with corpses was a cultural barrier for women originally entering and advancing in the field:

Yes, I feel that those autopsies constitute this bottleneck that many women don't get through. It demands a certain attitude and perhaps this kind of— for men—typical showing off that they don't feel anything [laughs]. This isn't very typical for women, I think. (#1)

The emotional reaction of women students to the anatomy lab experience constitutes one of the main reasons that women are not able to do as well as the male students:

And this [emotional reaction] you can recognize with women students when there are those autopsy demonstrations. Well, the women clearly react to those emotionally, and they have a hard time somehow getting to work. (#1)

Autopsies are work in which the culture of the medical profession suggests that men are needed. As indicated above, autopsy work and its gendered character constitute the master status of the pathologist. Although autopsies might be seen by outsiders as "dirty work," within the professional group of pathologists this work has been surrounded with a certain aura of status and competence. This competence has been defined in both physical and emotional terms, and it resembles the skills assumed to be required for doing surgery (Fox 1992; Katz 1999; Cassell 2000). Some of the informants referred to the hard physical work needed for doing autopsies, which was considered work not appropriate for a woman—a view the women did not embrace:

In the autopsies, there's always an assistant present to do the hardest work and the technically most demanding tasks—sawing and such—so we don't have to saw bones. I could easily learn how to do it, though. (#6)

Ergonomically the dissection tables and such—well, they're designed for larger persons than, for instance, me. So that obviously the work environment, in this respect, fits men better. But in my opinion, there's nothing in the work itself—well, there's nothing that a woman would stand less than a man would. (#7)

Others referred to the work in more emotional terms, as being seen as more appropriate for their male colleagues:

And the general notion is also that doing the autopsies don't quite fit women, and I realize, for example, that now in my everyday work I haven't had autopsy duty for many months. The chief physician, who does the duty list, obviously he—he certainly doesn't do it consciously—but my name is always missing from it [laughs]. I don't really object, of course, but I really could do them. (#1)

But even those women pathologists who were mainly doing microscopy felt after a time at this type of work that it was difficult to go back to the hands-on skills of their trade:

I think it's that the autopsies somehow scare women. Many men don't like it either. . . . It's not very nice work, and I have observed that to do it you have to do it without emotion—coldly—and you have to do it all the time. So now that I haven't done autopsies for a long time, I feel I have this barrier to starting to do it again. In fact, I realized this when I'd been here a couple of years and one of my colleagues asked me to do autopsies for her during her summer vacation. Then I had nightmares from them, and somehow it was surprisingly difficult. When you do it all the time, you get used to it. (#7)

As a way of countering the masculine image of autopsy, the informants constructed a shared image of the female skills needed in microscopy. They tended to portray themselves as more fit than their male colleagues in microscopy. It was argued that women had a sense of thoroughness, order, and detail, they were handy and diligent, attributes that were presented as functional requirements for professional work in pathology. This rhetoric surrounding women's propensity for detailed observation and craft-type work is a discursive strategy of *gender inclusion* presented by women pathologists themselves so as to legitimate their professional competence in the internal differentiation of work in pathology (see also Witz 1992). This gendered assignment was given chiefly by middle-aged women pathologists, a fact that might be related to their seniority in the laboratory, while the younger women were still given a variety of tasks:

> This is also a field where one needs precision, where women in general are better. Hard-working, careful workers—that's the work image of a pathologist, and it generally fits women. (#2)

> Autopsies are not that nice, but this microscopy is clean indoor work that in my opinion fits well with women's way of thinking. And there's also this in microscopy you have to consider the visual aspect, and what you have learned previously, and the movements of the hands—and coordinate all those three and draw a conclusion. This suits women's way of thinking very well. (#8)

The informants, who were all women pathologists, were all defending gender equality but still defended their position with a qualification that being women implied that they were the carriers of the craft skills of their occupational group:

> There are no gender differences, or else women are even better than men doctors, perhaps more conscientious and in a way more exact in dissection— taking a sample—well, women somehow examine the sample more carefully and then take another sample from the right place, are more exact, note more exactly where it's taken from and how it looks. And this preexamination is more exact. (#5)

And another woman argued:

> I can imagine that a woman can do [work in pathology] better than men because women have this kind of stamina—they can stand to sit. But then

when one thinks about pathologists in general, there are no gender differences. (#6)

Hence, though autopsy work was the master status of the pathologists and this status was male gendered, microscopy was portrayed in female-gendered terms by the women pathologists. Such a description of the skills for doing a good job in microscopy legitimated women's tasks in the field and constituted a strategy of gender inclusion.

## DOING THE WORK: THE GENDERED DIVISION OF LABOR

In the women's accounts of work in pathology, there appeared two types of reasons for the internal differentiation by gender. These two mechanisms can be characterized as *gender inclusion* and *gender casting*. As a social mechanism they have the same function: they constitute a mechanism of interpersonal control, although they differ in the extent that women have control over the definition of the situation. As shown above, gender inclusion is a discursive strategy whereby women pathologists legitimate their tasks within a certain jurisdiction of medical work. Gender casting here means a process whereby somebody projects someone of the opposite gender into a particular identity or role type. The concept is an elaboration of the term *alter casting* introduced by Weinstein and Deutschberger (1963) to account for the processual character of interpersonal interaction and identity construction neglected in Goffman's (1959) original contribution. By means of gender casting, women pathologists were defined by their male colleagues as being in a certain niche of work. Women's traditional gender attributes and tasks—taking care of children—were used as a rationale for delegating to women certain types of work in pathology. Women pathologists were assumed to have a certain affinity to the tissues or, in the words of Keller (1983), "a feeling for the organism." So, the tissue samples not only of children but of women patients were considered part of women pathologists' gender-specific domain. One woman who had just entered the field observed:

Yes, it's a quite interesting phenomenon that there clearly exists men's work and women's work. Really it's quite evident. It appears that, well—although, I have not specialized yet—I'm being given certain types of work. I think it's quite funny that it seems that women have to look, for example, at cell samples, and it seems as if children's genetic samples for some reason belong to women although [the samples] are already on a glass in the microscope. It's funny in some way. (#1)

Another woman who had worked in the field for a longer time reflected:

Somehow children's autopsies and generally all work related to children are handed over to women. There's this joke that children belong to women even if the children are dead. (#3)

She was echoed by a third:

Certain specimens—children's specimens—tend to come to women pathologists readily. It's been said to me that it's been the custom for women pathologists to examine implants and embryos. (#5)

Work on dissected tissues from children was a skill added to women's general medical expertise. Although emotional work is a skill attributed to or adopted by women working in general practice, as noted by Brooks (1998), this skill was assumed to make women pathologists more suited than their male colleagues to undertake work with children's tissues. It was assumed that women had the intimate knowledge and appropriate "feeling for the organism" (Keller 1983) because the dissected tissues were children's.

But attributing sex roles to organisms is lore that prevails in medical textbooks, as eminently shown by Martin (1991) in her review of how medical science has constructed a romance between the egg and the sperm to account for the process of fertilization and reproduction. This same kind of lore based on a stereotypical female-mother-caring role is carried over to the everyday work of pathology, with children's tissues considered objects-as-subjects needing the emotional support and caring concern of a mother-pathologist. Here the very normative basis of pathology is transgressed. In general, pathology's mandate in medicine enters when the body has been classified as matter. Nevertheless, fatal disease but also subjectivity were inscribed in children's tissues. Thus the cultural and normative expectations related to children's and women's status in society have impinged on work pursued in pathology and have been reproduced in the kind of medical work done by women pathologists.

However, women pathologists were not merely passive "victims" of gender casting that assigned them certain tasks. They were themselves contributing to the general medical lore by constructing certain female-gendered attributes as being part of the professional competence to form an exact expert opinion by means of microscopy. As shown in the preceding section, here an appeal to women's traditional skills for handicraft and precision was presented as making women particularly suited for the modern research-type work in pathology. Women were characterized by their innate gender skills as more fit for the work with tissue samples. Although visualization of disease as inscribed in the tissue was the primary craft skill of a pathologist, the informants thought that women had a special sense of thoroughness, order, and detail. They were also handy and diligent, attributes that they saw as functional requirements for professional work in pathology.

Hence, gender casting was the mechanism whereby women pathologists' work was limited by their male colleagues to certain areas, whereas gender inclusion, as defined by the women themselves, not only legitimated their role in microscopy but also defined the very essence of the professional skills perceived to be needed in that kind of specialist work.

## CONCLUSIONS

This chapter has described the internal differentiation of work within the specialty of pathology, and in particular how gender is embedded in the social definition of the special skills required for certain tasks. The biological raw material of the human body constitutes the concrete objective of the work of the pathologist. The chapter has provided an account of how women pathologists in Finland define the qualities needed for the basic tasks in pathology—autopsy work and visualization of disease through microscopy. Doing autopsies still forms the master status of this occupational group, although today the main task of pathologists is to provide clinicians with expert opinions about tissue samples from live patients who are screened for or have had or will have surgery for some ailment or disease. The task is more often to confirm the normality of such samples than to diagnose pathology.

Autopsy work is the master status of pathologists and this status has a male-gendered character, whereas microscopy is contextualized in female-gendered terms by the women pathologists themselves. Microscopy requires a "microscopic gaze" (Atkinson 1995), which is a way of visualizing the character of the tissue samples. To see the normal or the pathological in the tissue requires a shared knowledge and common concepts. Routine cases are done alone, whereas the diagnosis in a more problematic case is a result of a working consensus of the team. Microscopy is portrayed as requiring precision and stamina, a sense for order and details. These essential craft skills of the trade are associated with female skills.

There are two mechanisms of "doing gender" (West and Zimmerman 1987) in pathology. These mechanisms not only construct the gendered tasks but provide a legitimation for the internal division of labor by gender in pathology. The mechanisms of the construction of gender-specific tasks within pathology are *gender casting* and *gender inclusion*. In gender casting women are assigned certain tasks by men within the division of labor in pathology, tasks that are a priori considered to belong to women. Such a gendered task is the study of dissected tissue samples taken from children, a task considered "natural" for a woman pathologist. The emotional work done by women in society is added to the medical skills of women pathologists. In this sense, women pathologists have, in the eyes of their male colleagues, a certain "feeling for the organism," a gender-specific competence that renders certain tasks "natural" for them. This kind of gender asset has been valorized by women physicians themselves in primary-care specialties (West 1993; Brooks 1998; Riska and Wegar 1995; Pringle 1998; Le Feuvre 1999) and has been a kind of mother attribute given to token women in management positions (Kanter 1977). An attitude and image of blending in and almost concealing the feminine attributes has, on the other hand, been found to be the strategy among token women professionals in surgery (Conley 1998; Cassell 2000) and in many male-dominated professions (Sheppard 1989). This was not the strategy adopted by women pathologists.

Instead gender inclusion was the strategy they used as they constructed a legitimation for their gender-specific skills in microscopy. Here they also used essentialist arguments related to women's feminine skills, but these skills are viewed in instrumental rather than emotional terms: precision, diligence, endurance, a sense of order, a propensity for detailed observation are considered to constitute the core of the ethos and the visual skills required of a pathologist. The same feminine attributes have been recognized as uniquely feminine by women working in female-dominated, lower-level white-collar occupations—for example, in a study of Finnish female insurance clerks (Korvajärvi 1997:74). The lower-level white-collar women identified these attributes qualifying them for routine tasks as the degrading and dead-end aspects of their work. By contrast, the women pathologists interviewed in this study valorized the same attributes as the essence of professionalism and prerequisite for professional competence in the work they were doing.

# 8

## Women's Challenge of Medicine

### *A Revolution From Within or Outside Medicine?*

### INTRODUCTION

In the introductory chapter the question was raised as to whether women physicians represent a potential humanistic and holistic approach to medicine and a group that will head the rest of the profession toward a substantial change in the way medicine is practiced, or whether women have been relegated to a marginal and "proletarianized" position in the profession, which at the same time indicates their lack of power to change even their own conditions of work. The question can also be raised in narrower and more feminist terms: Can women change medicine? How can they? Can they best do it from *within* or from *outside*? What has been women physicians' part in the feminist challenges of medicine in the three settings examined in this volume?

Chapters 3, 4, and 5 showed that the pioneering women physicians were assigned and committed to taking care of women's and children's health needs in the three settings. As women physicians became full-fledged members of the medical profession, the women's issues gradually faded as women and children were no longer the sole constituency of women physicians.

In the late 1960s and 1970s, the second wave of the women's movement gave women's health issues a new salience in many Western societies: feminists began to challenge medicine as a social institution and pointed to the gender-biased medical knowledge and practices pursued by its predominantly male physicians. How did women physicians relate to these developments?

Much of the field of women's health as a feminist issue and movement have been colored by the U.S. debate and developments. This literature has tended to remain silent on the role of women physicians, and in fact the gender of the individual physician has been less at issue than the male-dominated paradigm of medicine that has been assumed to be used by physicians regardless of gender. For some feminists, women physicians

117

have been easier to accept if it is shown that they occupy a subordinate position in the medical profession and thus share the characteristics of most other women (see Pringle 1998:2). In such a case it has been assumed that there is a common female culture uniting women as clients and providers of health care. In this debate a feminist-standpoint theory of women's interests and basis for acting has been predominant. The basic assumption of the radical feminists in the women's health movement in the 1970s was that women were subordinated and oppressed by medicine and the state, both of which were viewed as serving patriarchal interests and reproducing the patriarchal gender order. This notion has been less prevalent in the other two settings examined here—the Scandinavian countries and Russia, where a liberal and a socialist feminist stance, respectively, have served as the basis for issues concerning women's health and health care.

Since the feminist criticism of the medical profession and subsequently a whole genre of sociological studies on women's health emerged within the U.S. debate, it is important to review here, first, the feminist challenges of medicine in the U.S. context. In the U.S. and British feminist debate, women's health has been presented as a generic concept, and the feminist issues as applicable universally (see, e.g., Gray 1998; Doyal 1983). It is the argument of this chapter that the construct "women's health" has served an important ideological function in local or national debates but cannot be used as a generic concept for comparative research purposes since there is no clear definition of what kind of services should or even could fall under such a generic concept. "Women's health" agendas are generally directly linked to the gender order and health care system of a country and have to be analyzed within that country's cultural, social, and political context. This chapter will therefore examine women's challenge of medicine separately for each context.

The following sections will first present the general debate on women's health as a feminist issue in the U.S. context. In the United States, women's health became a rallying concept for feminists who wanted to change medicine from the outside. However, recent U.S. developments have witnessed a transformation of women's health concerns due not only to commercial ventures in the area, but also to new professional advocates within medicine. It is interesting to compare and contrast this development with that in the Scandinavian societies, where women's health concerns have been integrated into existing welfare state policies. Here the policies pursued seem more to have followed a strategy of changing medicine from within established institutions. The latter societies are by no means homogeneous in this respect, as this chapter will show. Denmark witnessed a strong women's movement and a concomitant women's health movement in the 1970s. By contrast, in Norway, Sweden, and Finland—particularly in the latter two countries—there has been a professional dominance over the issues related to women's health needs and a weak lay organization for alternative health services for women.

Since the 1990s, the U.S. and Scandinavian situations seem to have come closer to each other in the sense that an equal rights or a liberal feminist perspective and a group of professional reformers within medicine are articulating the needs in the field of women's health. One reason for this feature is the demise of a laywomen's health movement, but also an increasing differentiation of women's health issues. The narrow and specialized concerns involved in women's health issues in the 1990s not only resulted in a medicalization of the issues, but also in a call for technical solutions, inviting a variety of experts to solve women's health issues. Since Russia/Soviet Union has been outside this debate, the focus will mainly be on U.S. and Scandinavian developments.

## FEMINIST CHALLENGES OF MEDICINE IN THE UNITED STATES

The purpose of this section is to examine the feminist challenges of medicine in U.S. society and what kind of strategies to change medicine have been adopted in the U.S. setting since the 1970s. Two questions have guided the following presentation of the transformation of the concerns for women's health in the United States from the late 1960s to the late 1990s. First, over the past three decades, what kind of issues have been advocated by the feminist critics? Second, what have been the roles of women physicians and laywomen who have promoted women's health issues during each decade? The movement has gone through three stages: The first stage was the rise of feminist health collectives in the 1970s and a broader cultural critique of U.S. medicine from a feminist viewpoint. The second stage was the decline of feminist women's health centers and the co-optation of the issue of women's health by the private medical market in the 1980s. The third stage consists of the endeavors in the 1990s pursued by a group of professional reformers—feminist, academic women physicians—locating the knowledge and practice of women's health not only within medicine but to be pursued by professionals: "women's health physicians."

### The Women's Health Movement of the 1970s and 1980s

The U.S. women's health movement in the 1970s was not the first time U.S. women became collectively concerned with health issues pertaining to women. The earlier movement spanned a period from the mid-1870s to the late 1890s. The issues of both movements seem, however, to have been the same: a challenge of the medical knowledge of regular doctors, an interest in women's control over their bodies as part of a larger demand of control of women in society, lay and self-help activities, a sense of shared feminist collectivism, and women physicians' engagement to advance women's health. Historians have provided ample documentation of the earlier phase of the women's health movement in the United States (see, e.g., Morantz 1977a, 1977b; Morantz-Sanchez 1985; Apple 1990). They have related its emergence to the rise of the middle-class woman and her quest for economic and political rights, all of which have to be seen against the backdrop of the larger social change created by a rapid industrialization and urbanization in the United States. Less is known about the subsequent development of the women's health movement of the 1970s, although an interest in the issue seems to have emerged lately (e.g., Thomas 1993; Ruzek and Becker 1999). In this literature, the endeavors of laywomen have been in focus, whereas the role of women physicians has been largely invisible.

The beginnings of the women's health movement in the early 1970s has been eminently documented by Ruzek (1978) in her detailed account of the ideological issues, the politics and collective actions, and the women's health-related organizations and service centers up to the mid-1970s. As Ruzek shows, the concrete steps toward an organization around the issue of women's health began with a discussion group on "Women and Their Bodies" at a large women's conference in Boston in the spring of 1969 (ibid.:32). Afterwards, a group of women in Boston did research and wrote papers on women's health and began to organize courses on the topic. The mimeographed notes and papers were bound together into the first edition of the self-help manual *Our Bodies, Ourselves* (Boston Women's Health Book Collective 1973), which came to have an unexpected, catalytic role in creating an avalanche of response among feminist-oriented women across the country.

The rise of the women's health movement did not, however, appear overnight with the publication of *Our Bodies, Ourselves*. Instead, the movement has to be seen as part of a variety of social movements that were germane to the U.S. society of the 1960s: the civil rights movement, the consumer movement, the peace and draft-resistance movement, and the emerging second-wave feminist movement. As women supported and/or participated in these movements, parallel issues relating to their status as women in the United States came gradually to the surface (Thorne 1975). For example, the consumer movement criticized the dominant auto, tobacco, and drug industries for not considering the safety of their products for the consumer. This was a time when the drug industry was seriously criticized for harming women's health (e.g., thalidomide treatments were debated in Europe) and physicians came to be portrayed as the prolonged arm of the capitalist and patriarchal order that controlled and subjugated women as bodies and selves. A concrete case against the drug industry was Barbara Seaman's (1969) investigation of the safety of oral contraceptives published as a book, *The Doctors' Case Against the Pill*. The book created a debate on women's health that culminated in a hearing in Congress on the safety of the contraceptive pill in 1970.

The main argument of the various branches of the women's movement in the 1970s was that women did not have control over their bodies and their own health (Zimmerman 1987:443). The radical feminists in the women's health movement perceived biomedicine as a hegemonic male-generated construct practiced by a male-dominated medical profession. Medicine was portrayed as part of a larger social and political control by men over women. One of the major goals of the movement was to expose the social structures that shape women's health and to reclaim the ownership of the knowledge and treatment of women's health, especially as related to reproduction. The major task was first to demystify the female body by redefining it in nonpathological terms, and then to organize health care around a new knowledge and model (Fee 1977). The body-consciousness-raising activities had a crucial role in the women's health movement because these activities were aimed at raising women's feminist and political consciousness in order to change the gender system in society. The health collectives were a means to this consciousness raising and empowerment of women at the grassroots level. But some saw in women's challenge of medicine the beginning of a much larger change and restructuring of U.S. medicine. For example, in her review of the U.S. women's health movement, Marieskind (1975:221) foresaw in this movement a "potential revolutionary force" in its demand for restructuring of the total health care system and a redefinition of health care, not only for women but for the whole population. Its greatest contribution, she argued, was, in "a change in the consciousness of men and women freed from the binding roles of domination and submission" (ibid.:222).

But as Elizabeth Fee (1977) reminds us, there were not only radical and socialist feminists among the women's health advocates and activists in the 1970s but liberal feminists as well. The liberal feminists accepted the basic structure of the existing health care system and demanded women's access to health care as a right and as part of their broader quest for equality. The demands were phrased in a consumerist model—more and different kinds of services for women and women's access to positions of power in medicine as physicians, administrators, and policymakers. As will be shown later in this chapter, it is this group of women's health advocates that seem to have gained strength in the 1990s.

In the 1970s, feminists did not turn to women physicians as their allies, nor did women physicians as a group emerge as solidary supporters of the lay feminist cause of changing medicine from the outside. This has, however, to be looked at in the light of the weak representation that women at this time had in the U.S. medical profession. In 1970, women constituted merely 7 percent of the physicians in the United States, only one percentage point higher than in 1900. Although individual women physicians were drawn to the causes of the contemporary women's health movement, their involvement as a professional group remained largely invisible. Their own professional opportunities in U.S. medicine were, however, much advanced at this time since U.S. medical schools had adopted affirmative-action policies.

The challenge from the outside came from laywomen organized as lay-run feminist health collectives that served as an alternative to the hierarchical pattern of male medicine. The new model was called the "well-woman's" model or feminist health-service model, and it challenged the unnecessary medicalization of women's bodies. By 1973, there were around one hundred feminist health clinics, and by 1975 altogether 280 women's health centers and women's health organizations provided health services to women (Ruzek 1978; Thomas 1993). These clinics were run by lay volunteers, who offered instructions in gynecological self-examination, preventive health care, pregnancy testing, family planning, and pregnancy and abortion counseling. The emphasis was on self-help—laywomen assisting other women and passing on to them their experience-based knowledge. If professional medical help was needed, a woman-friendly physician who enjoyed the trust of the lay collective was called in. A good example of such a lay practice was an illegal feminist abortion collective in Chicago, through whose efforts eleven thousand abortions were performed from 1969 to 1973 (Bart 1987).

The Supreme Court decision legalizing abortion in 1973 resulted in an official recognition of the need for counseling on family planning and abortion. For the feminist health centers this legislation posed a dilemma: On the one hand, it was now possible to get the much-needed economic support; but, on the other hand, the federal rules imposed new structures and procedures alien to the very ideology of the centers. Many feminists distrusted the federal agencies and feared an external control and distortion of the objectives of the movement and therefore refrained from any involvement with the federal agencies. Other women's health centers found the external support a much-needed economic asset to their shoestring operation but soon found out that the original structures and goals of the organization were transformed (see also Broom 1991:106–7).

In a case study of an U.S. feminist health clinic and the changes in the organization and services it underwent from 1972 to 1980, Morgen (1986) shows that the federal requirements imposed a social-service and provider-client orientation instead of the previous social-change and feminist orientation of the health collective. The external public funding put new demands on the organization, and a paid staff and a director had to be appointed. The new, paid personnel gave rise to a hierarchical structure as opposed to the volunteer and collective decision-making of the past. Furthermore, the center had to diversify its staff by race and class and to endorse a more activist conception of feminism than the abstract feminist principles embraced by the middle-class volunteers running the collective at its inception. This development leads Morgen (ibid.:208–9) to conclude that the external public funding actually forced an implementation of the more visionary objectives that the collective had set as its goal originally.

The original women's health centers established in the early 1970s had began as centers providing well-woman care and self-help as a way to empower women in the health care market. A decline of the feminist health services organizations began in the 1980s. The social organization for women's health did not vanish but was transformed by new promoters and private agencies. In the 1980s, women's health became a service that other health care organizations began to integrate into their offerings to women as health care consumers.

The first to adopt the original preventive and holistic aspect of the women's health movement were the Health Maintenance Organizations (HMOs). It was a sincere effort by many laywomen, attracted by the message of the women's health movement, to integrate the same concerns into the consumer-run, nonprofit health care delivery of the early HMOs (Looker 1993). By mid-1980s, the original endeavors of the HMOs had been subjugated to the wave of corporatization of the health care market in the United States.

The second to adopt the women's health issues were health care organizations in the private market. There was a growing commercial interest in women's health since it was recognized that women were the primary consumers of health care. In the commercial cloning of the women's health centers, the terminology of the original movement was used with profit but stripped of its feminist ideology and message of the empowerment of women (Looker 1993; Thomas 1993). However, Zimmerman and Hill (2000:780) suggest that women are receiving increasing levels of preventive care as a result of managed-care plans.

A new obstacle for the activities of the feminist health centers was the antichoice movement with its radical attacks on women's health centers. The antiabortionist and New Right movement not only waged ideological warfare with but also posed a physical threat to the practice of the women's health centers of whatever stripe.

## The Issue of Women's Health in the 1990s: The Professional Advocacy for Women's Health

The demise of the original women's health movement as a grassroots movement and feminist endeavor was a fact in the United States by the early 1990s: of the one hundred feminist health centers in existence in 1973, only twenty-four were still in operation in 1993 (Thomas 1993). The commercial interest in well-woman care has expanded, and hospital-based women's health centers have emerged. In the 1990s, a renewed interest in women's health was shown by various professional women's groups at the federal level, to be seen in the promotion of women's health concerns by feminist women physicians in academe. Two types of issues have been advanced: first, federally funded research on women's health and, second, establishment of a curriculum in women's health in U.S. medical schools and efforts to create an interdisciplinary specialty in women's health.

In the mid-1980s, the concern over the lack of knowledge about women's diseases and health patterns resulted in a number of concrete activities. Political action on the issue was pushed by lobbying groups such as Women's Health Action Mobilization and Women's Action Coalition, but the concrete suggestions for research on women's health were laid out in the Public Health Service Task Force on Women's Health Issues in 1985 (Auerbach and Figert 1995:117). It resulted in the policy of the National Institutes of Health (NIH), in operation since 1987, of encouraging the inclusion of women in clinical scientific trials. Nevertheless, the guidelines were found not to have been followed consistently, and in 1990 the NIH responded by establishing an Office of Research on Women's Health, the task of which was to coordinate research on women's health and promote biomedical career opportunities for women. Concrete measures for promoting research on women's health were solidified in the project launched by NIH under the heading of Women's Health Initiative in 1991. This was a fourteen-year study on women's health with a budget of $625 million in 1991, and secured in the future by the NIH Revitalization Amendments in 1993 (Auerbach and Figert 1995; *Science* 1995). It was not a coincidence that the first woman to serve as the director of NIH, Bernadine Healy, was also appointed in 1991. But the support for the new endeavors in the area of women's health came from a larger political coalition of women—the women's caucus in the Congress and the Senate, who already in 1990 had introduced the Women's Health Equity Act (Shumaker and Smith 1994) In 1994, the Office of Women's Health was established at the Centers for Disease Control (CDC) in Atlanta to integrate women's health as part of CDC's prevention efforts. In 1997, $500 million of CDC money targeted women's health issues. In 1996 and 1997, the Office of Research on Women's Health of the NIH held a series of national scientific and public hearings to revise the agenda for women's health research. The final report, *Agenda for Research on Women's Health for the 21st Century*, provides a list of recommendations for the implementation of research findings on women's health and a list of women's health needs (Pinn 1999).

The other agenda that emerged in the 1990s was the claiming of the knowledge about women's health by feminist women physicians active in academe. The knowledge was to be holistic and interdisciplinary and, as one of the early promoters of a specialty in women's health (Johnson and Dawson 1990:224) phrased it, "Women's health is being defined as a specific body of knowledge and expertise that permits the comprehensive care of women." The field was launched as an interdisciplinary primary-care specialty with a special focus on women:

> Woman-centered care means creating a system around women's specific health needs *and* women's styles of interacting. Within the current paradigm, lesbians, women of color, poor women, and older women rarely receive the level of care appropriate to their needs. (Johnson and Hoffman 1993:117)

The endeavor in the 1990s to create a specialty in women's health departs from the belief in institutional change by means of laywomen. At issue is no longer a quest for a broader challenge of economic and political institutions presented under the slogan "The Private Is Political." Instead, the new knowledge production on women's health has been integrated into the institutional structure of biomedicine, where the women's health agenda is promoted by a cadre of professional reformers—women physicians teaching in medical schools. Women's health has become a legitimate field of the medical curriculum. As the president of the Association of American Medical Colleges recently stated in a leading article in *Academic Medicine*, the journal of the association: "Women's health is now a well recognized and growing medical discipline." He concludes: "So it's encouraging to recognize that so many initiatives are now in place to accelerate the pace of progress toward a truly equitable and unbiased health care system" (Cohen 1999:1226).

The new specialty of women's health can be viewed as a professional project of a cohort of women physicians who present themselves as the professional advocates of women's health and as defenders of women's interests in medicine. Nevertheless, these professional reformers of medicine view themselves as part of the broader women's and women's health movement. For example, Bernadine Healy, the editor of the *Journal of Women's Health*, argues that the current stage can be equated with a third suffrage movement:

> The emphasis on women's health that we are witnessing now is a form of suffrage movement, for women to focus on their quality of life, that by necessity grew out of two earlier movements. (1995:219)

The initiatives in the academic settings have been endorsed at the federal level. In October 1996, the Office of Women's Health of the Public Health Service Office established the first model centers that would provide integrated and comprehensive women's health services to women across the country. The first generation of six centers was located at Allegheny University of the Health Sciences in Philadelphia, Magee-Women's Hospital in Pittsburgh, the University of California at San Francisco, the University of Pennsylvania in Philadelphia, and Yale University in New Haven. These centers were proposed to "serve as one-stop shopping models targeted to the unique health care needs of women." A year later a second generation of six "National Centers of Excellence" was established, and in 1998 a third generation of such centers, bringing the number up to eighteen.

## Underlying Values Promoting Women's Health as a Professional Project

Underlying the initiatives in women's health pursued in the United States over the past three decades are three specific values related to the U.S. setting: *consumerism, health as an individualized concern,* and the alleged *gender qualities of women physicians.*

First, in the U.S. feminist health movement, there has been an underlying, populist distrust of big capital and big government and their potential capacity to control women's decisions and lives. Instead, women's interests have been located in a decentralized organization of health care—feminist health collectives or a competitive market—which are assumed to optimize women's capacity to have control over their own decisions about treatments and their bodies. Hence, the women physicians' current claims for a medical specialty in women's health care have been framed within a market-based organization of health care. A central claim has been that certain marginalized groups—poor, old, black, and lesbian women—have not been provided the services that meet their needs as *consumers in the health care market.* The new type of physician—"the woman's health physician"—is envisioned to "maintain a respectful, collaborative, and consumer-oriented approach, with women as their health care partners" (Johnson and Dawson 1990:223) and to encourage women patients to "maintain informed responsibility for their own health care choices" (Johnson and Hoffman 1993:117). Hence, women's health needs are envisioned as met within a market-based system of health care and by means of a reform of medicine by forces within medicine.

Second, *health as an individualized concern* has become a predominant feature in the 1990s, not only in the United States but also in most Western countries. In the early 1980s, Crawford (1980) drew attention to the new focus on health in the United States. He called the new feature "healthism," which he saw as a personal preoccupation with health and an increasing emphasis on the individual's responsibility for his or her health. Wagner (1997) has developed this theme further and calls the preoccupation with personal health in the 1990s the New Puritanism and New Temperance. Wagner argues that the personal preoccupation with one's own health and the emergence of health as a virtue have individualized and depoliticized health as a social issue (see also Crawford 1984). Health is viewed as a personal and moral concern rather than a public health issue framed by gendered and economic structures. In this sense, Parsons's (1979) classic essay on health as a special value and an individual responsibility and concern in the United States has received a new salience.

The shift in the locus of responsibility is also reflected in the area of women's health. In the 1970s, women's health was raised as a public issue by the lay advocates within the women's health movement, and a collective sense and collective responsibility for women's health emerged within that movement. The 1990s has witnessed a change in the definition of health from a political to a private issue—it has taken the form of an individualized concern and an individual project. Such an individualized view is also promoted by the women's health organizations' reaching individual women through the electronic media. Women can reach various self-help groups and access information about their health from a variety of websites. At these Internet connections the biomedical discourse speaks with equal authority as a discourse of alternative medicine. As Ruzek and Becker (1999:8) observe, in today's virtual world a variety of groups claim to speak for women. Their own surfing of U.S. websites harvested 223 national women's health organizations serving as women's health advocates.

It would be wrong to conclude that there is no interest in women's health in the 1990s. More women than ever think today about their health as they pursue aerobics, jogging, and vegetarian diets, explore their risks for ovarian and breast cancer, and change their lifestyle and health behavior accordingly. At issue are different types of politics. There is no longer a unitary, political women's health movement but instead individual and group actions focused on very special and narrow issues. For example, since the mid-1990s there has been a breast cancer movement among U.S. women, a movement that is ideologically fragmented into diverse strands (Klawiter 1999).

The remaining feminist initiatives have focused on specific issues, such as rape, incest, eating disorders, drug dependency, battered women. Although important for women's quality of life, the focus of these issues is on individual women and individual men. Hence, as the feminist critique has unfolded, it has transformed itself from a critique of patriarchy to a moralistic crusade against violence committed by individual men against individual women. This moralistic approach or discourse is related to the changes in the way that health is defined in the 1990s (Wagner 1997). As Zimmerman and Hill (2000:777) in their review of the U.S. feminist consumer model of health care note, the underlying notion of personal responsibility offers merely an illusion of control because in fact there is no power and equity for women if they are held responsible for gendered conditions they cannot alter or avoid, e.g., poor working conditions, rape, domestic violence.

Third, the transformation of health from a collective to an individual concern is conducive to the emergence of the current claim to women's health by the professional reformers among academic women physicians. The individualistic approach to women's health issues matches the medical approach represented by the academic interest in women's health in the 1990s. Historically, the woman physician's role as a partner with the woman patient has been a claim that the women physicians have presented as a legitimation for their quest for a domain of their own within the U.S. medical profession. Such an inclusionary strategy was early a device for legitimating their position within the male-dominated profession, as shown in Chapter 3 (Drachman 1984; Morantz-Sanchez 1985; More 1999). A central feature of the U.S. discussion about women as providers of health care has been the conviction that *women physicians have certain gender qualities* and that they differ from their male counterparts, a claim that is still advanced today (e.g., Ulstad 1993). The woman physician is presented by the representatives of this view as a repository of female values and virtues and a benevolent medical practitioner who promotes a holistic and woman-oriented approach in medicine, as opposed to the allegedly narrow view of the male members of the profession. Underlying this essentialist conviction is the view that women—whether as patients or providers—have some truth claims about women's health.

## WOMEN'S HEALTH MOVEMENTS: A MISSING FEMINIST MOVEMENT IN THE SCANDINAVIAN COUNTRIES?

The tide of social reformism that spurred women's involvement in charity work and public health in the United States at the turn of the twentieth century also had a comparable expression in the Scandinavian context. But women's political rights were recognized earlier in the Scandinavian countries than in the United States (in 1920): women gained the right to participate in parliamentary elections in Finland in 1906, in Norway in 1913, in Denmark in 1915, and in Sweden (an exception) in 1921 (Skard and Haavio-Mannila 1985:38). The early integration of women into the political system in Scandinavia imprinted a special profile on women's political activities. The feminist agendas related to health and social services were voiced through formal political channels. Rantalaiho (1997), in her analysis of the development of women's citizenship in the Scandinavian welfare states, argues that the discourse of gender difference in the early twentieth century channeled women into separate women's organizations within existing political parties. Within their gender-specific niches in the political system women became the experts on their "own" areas and represented their own female constituencies. Women politicians worked over party boundaries to advance women's issues, a legacy that has been called "state feminism." In its contemporary expression, it is a political strategy that uses the state as a defender of gender equality and women's issues rather than viewing the state, as the radical feminists do, as an oppressor of women (ibid.:23).

The post–World War II scene in Scandinavia, particularly in Sweden, has been characterized by policies promoting gender equality and a model of the family based on the dual-earner household (Huber and Stephens 2000:337). For women the public discourse on "wage-worker motherhood" has implied a normalization of women's paid employment in Scandinavia. This view on women has been followed by an acknowledgement of parenthood as part of the worker citizens' responsibilities, and equality policies have been used as the ideological means to construct the Scandinavian welfare state. The parental leave system for parents of children under age one, the availability of municipal child care for children under six, and legislation (e.g., in Finland and Sweden) allowing parents to shorten their daily working hours are measures that have improved women's position in the labor market—and in the family. The combination of wage work and children is not perceived as an obstacle by Scandinavian women, a circumstance that leads many to opt for professional careers, thus explaining the high percentage of women in medicine.

While the gender-equality ideology permeates the view on women's position in Scandinavia, there is a discrepancy between this ideology and practice. As Dahlerup (1994:122) points out, "the sharing [of work between men and women] model" is the official ideology in the Scandinavian countries, the "double-burden-for-women model" is more often the practice. The Scandinavian welfare states are said to be based on a gender contract that harbors a "tacit gender compromise" (Rantalaiho 1997:27): women have the right to work but they still have the major responsibility for the family.

In contrast to U.S. developments in the 1970s, the second wave of the women's movement did not crystallize into a strong women's health movement in Norway, Sweden, and Finland in the 1970s and 1980s. This development relates to the differences in the way that women's health has been approached in the different contexts. In the U.S. context, women's health was in the 1970s viewed as an issue related to the body of the individual woman—her right to have control over her body and biological reproduction on her own terms. In a paradoxical way, the U.S. women's health movement has almost medicalized women's bodies by focusing on health services as a matter of the physiological body and sexuality. In the Scandinavian context, especially in Sweden and Finland, women's access to health services and the institutionalization of health services for women within the maternity care services have been part of public family policy. These endeavors are part of what Esping-Andersen (1996:14) calls the "social investment" or preventive approach in Scandinavian social policy. The values of universalism and equity have been the organizing principles of how services have been set up. Women's health issues have not been pursued as single issues but as part of the broader political agenda of labor unions and political parties. In this endeavor, women politicians have had a strategic role. The liberal feminist view, stressing gender equality and equal rights, has been the major strategy for securing health services to women.

A strong feminist health movement emerged as part of the second-wave feminist movement of the 1970s in Denmark. The emergence of a strong and independent feminist movement in Denmark has to be seen against the background of the economic situation and welfare-state policies adopted there in the 1970s. Denmark was hit by an economic recession and unemployment much earlier than the other Scandinavian countries, which experienced their crisis in the early 1990s. In addition, the financing of welfare services in Denmark has been mainly through taxation rather than via employer contribution as in the other Scandinavian countries. This has meant that service provisions have been more vulnerable to economic changes as well as to significant welfare cuts than in the other Scandinavian countries (Stephens 1996:54)

A group of women called Rødstrømperne—the Redstockings—constituted the core of the new women's movement in Denmark. The Redstockings, founded in the spring of 1970, were radical feminists who identified capitalism and patriarchy as the major oppressors of women (Dahlerup 1998). This was a cultural and political movement that took the form of a feminist counterculture, with no ambitions to establish itself at the national level or its goals on the national political agenda. Its central message was that "the private is political"; and feminist consciousness-raising and body consciousness took a central position in its activities. As an outgrowth of the feminist activities, a self-help manual *Kvinde kend din krop* (*Woman, Know Your Body*) emerged as a product of a feminist collective in 1975. This book was the Danish equivalent of the U.S. manual *Our Bodies, Ourselves* (Boston Women's Health Book Collective 1973). This alternative-knowledge production became a best-selling book, and it was brought out in two subsequent editions, in 1983 and in 1992.

*Kvinde kend din krop* (Vinder 1975) was launched as an alternative discourse on the body and gender, over against the normative femininity promoted by the male gaze and discourse of biomedicine. In a textual analysis of the three editions, Jørgensen (1993) found substantial differences in content and perspective. She argues that each edition is an example of the change that has taken place in women's own gaze on women during a twenty-year period. In each edition the understanding of femininity, the female body, and sex is constructed and reconstructed. The first edition of 1975 promotes an explicit radical feminist discourse (Vinder 1975). Women are perceived as victims of public control, power, and exploitation, and, according to the manual, feminist consciousness-raising is the major task of feminist groups. The second edition of 1983 (Vinder [1975] 1983) reflects the changes that had taken place in the feminist movement. The perspective of this edition is essentialist: Women's own experiences and femininity are valorized. The new theme is an acknowledgment of female sexuality as part of the female collective identity and experience. By contrast, in the 1992 edition (Vinder [1975] 1992), there is a strong individualistic undertone: Pluralism and differences among women are highlighted. At the same time new individual health issues are brought up—AIDS, incest, eating disorders, infertility. Sexuality is presented as an individual potential rather than as a heterosexual or lesbian collective identity, as it had been in the 1983 edition.

The Danish case illuminates a country with a strong women's health movement in the 1970s, which faded slightly after the demise of the Redstockings in mid-1980s. But the grassroots and antiestablishment character of the view on women's health has, however, remained a strong undercurrent in Denmark. The Danish feminist voices have been strong, and a critique of the establishment has continued to be part of the feminist activities. For example, while Swedish and Finnish women's organizations have been busy lobbying for integration of cancer or genetic screening into public health programs, among Danish feminists there has been hesitancy to embrace such endeavors. There has been a critique and a public hearing on the purported benefits for women of screening for breast cancer (see Petersson and Sørensen 1994), and Danish race laws and eugenic policies of the 1930s have been critically examined (Koch 1996). Furthermore, since the early 1970s birthing has been a widely debated issue and a strong lay organization promoting alternative birthing emerged (Haxthausen 1993).

In the 1990s, there was some convergence between U.S. and Scandinavian developments, although marked differences remain. As shown in

Chapter 4, in the Scandinavian countries the health professions can be called welfare-state occupations because their work, professional position, and legitimacy derive from their function in the welfare state (Elzinga 1990; Evertsson 2000). This has implied a standardization of services and setting of goals at the national level, a policy process that has very much been defined as "technical" and hence under the control of medical experts. "Women's interests" have been mainly treated as technical issues defined by experts so as to protect women from unscientific and commercial interests. More recently, the health technology assessment movement has focused on standards of "good" practice and demanded scientific evidence by means of controlled trials of the efficacy of most standard procedures and therapies used in current medical practice. The Swedish Council of Technology Assessment in Health Care has been particularly active in producing material drawn from "evidence-based medicine" for policymakers, especially in the area of women's health (e.g., a report on hysterectomy and on osteoporosis in 1995, on estrogen treatments in 1996, on routine ultrasound examination during pregnancy in 1998, on urinary incontinency and on IVF in 2000).

## CONCLUSIONS

In the 1970s, feminist scholars and health activists viewed biomedicine as codified knowledge that was part of the social order of men. In this sense, biomedicine was part of "abstract masculinity" (Hartsock 1983: 296-7), which rationalized the world of men but was separate from the "lifeworld of women" and their situated knowledge. Within feminist theory, the feminist-standpoint theory represented this stance in the 1970s: only women themselves possess true knowledge of womanly matters, because of their oppressed character and their specific life situation (Harding 1991:119; Hekman 1997). In the realm of medicine, this view meant that only women could have a correct perception and knowledge of their bodies, whereas the viewpoint of medical men was distorted, and their knowledge was part of the hegemonic discourse of masculine science.

The first wave of alternative-knowledge production within the women's health movements was based on the feminist-standpoint theory of knowledge. Women's own and shared experiences and experiential knowledge constituted the guidelines for the self-help endeavors of the early feminist health collectives (see also Taylor 1996). The emphasis was on lay knowledge and a shared experiential knowledge base on women's health by women themselves. The feminist-standpoint theory with its hegemonization of women—that is, the representation of a unitary concept of "woman's" interest—gradually became problematic, especially in the 1990s when the feminist debate began to emphasize the existence of differences among women (Hekman 1997).

The second wave of knowledge production rested on a perception that Harding (1991) has called "feminist empiricism" and others the "additive approach" (Andersen 1983). During the 1980s, there was an effort to generate new empirical knowledge about women's health. By adding new knowledge about women to existing medical knowledge, it was assumed that the medical sciences would become more objective and be used by physicians, regardless of gender, in a more informed way (see Rosser 1993).

While the production of new knowledge about women's health certainly filled a void in empirical knowledge about women's bodies, this endeavor did not prove to change the delivery of health services to women much. Professional reform of medicine by women physicians became a new strategy in the U.S. context: A new comprehensive medical knowledge base on women's health has been presented as a new specialty in U.S. medicine (Johnson and Hoffman 1993). In the 1990s, the professional reformers among academic women physicians adopted the agenda of women's health and reclaimed it as a professional concern. Armed with this scientific expertise, a special jurisdiction for women as patients in the U.S. health care system can be demarcated (see Abbott 1988). This jurisdiction is connected with a special provider and specialist—the women's health physician—and with the academic centers of women's health.

The demarcation of one area of medicine—women's health—can be seen as a professional strategy by U.S. academic women physicians to claim an exclusive but comprehensive knowledge of women's health. This can be seen as an inclusionary strategy: By establishing their own specialty in medicine with its own medical knowledge women's health physicians can create their own expertise and enhance their academic status and women's health as well. The specialty is to become an integrated part of the existing structure of U.S. medicine. Some of the female professional reformers have been defensive as they have countered what they have perceived as the "homogeneously antidoctor" stance of the women's health movement (see Cousins et al. 1994:409). Academic women physicians are in a problematic position vis-à-vis feminist lay health advocates: On the one hand, women physicians are part of medicine and a male-dominated profession but, on the other hand, they might feel different as a group from and marginal within the profession as a whole. Yet, the cadre of academic "women's health physicians" argues that gender differs in the practice of medicine. But as Pringle reminds us: "The issue is not whether women doctors are truly more caring than men but what can now be done with such claims" (1998:22).

Representatives of postmodern feminist thinking argue that concepts used in gender-related research are still based on essentialist notions.

According to a postmodern viewpoint, the definition of women's health is constructed on the binary notion of women and men, a notion that is based on unequally valued gender categories. It is argued that any construction of "women's health" takes as its departure point men's health as well as a biomedical model. As McCormick and her colleagues suggest: "Even though it does not use the word male or men's health, this is taken as the norm against which the definition of women's health is made" (1998:500). A desire for theoretical purity can, following its logical conclusion, lead a postmodernist to a nonadvocacy stance. Yet, McCormick and her collaborators (ibid.:503) encourage feminists to adopt a "strategic essentialist" stance (by which they mean that "woman" and "gender" should be used to achieve desired political ends for women and women's health) and at the same time remain aware of the limitations of current feminist theories about women and health. This is a position that Lorber (2000b) has identified as "gender-marked equity."

But do existing theoretical perspectives in the sociology of professions and feminist theory leave any promises for a more active role for women physicians in health care? In line with the theoretical approaches reviewed in Chapter 2, which addressed the underrepresentation of women in the higher ranks of the profession and in the organization of health care, these perspectives can also be used as *diagnostic perspectives* for suggesting a way to change women's position in the profession. According to the neo-Weberian approach, strengthening of the profession as a collective body would at the same time imply an improvement for all members of the profession, including women. A feminist strand of this perspective would encourage female professional subprojects to demarcate new areas and jurisdictions for women physicians (e.g., Witz 1992:48–50; Abbott 1988). The U.S. academic women physicians' movement for a specialty in women's health could be seen be an example of a gendered strategy of dual closure by employing demarcationary and inclusionary devices to define "women's health" as the jurisdiction of "women's health physicians." This discursive strategy was also evident in the accounts of women pathologists described in Chapter 7. Gender inclusion was the discursive strategy used by women pathologists when they constructed a legitimation for their gender-specific skills in microscopy.

A more traditional strategy has been to redefine gender attributes. According to this line of thinking, more affirmative values and role models in the gender and professional socialization of young women would result in changes in women's representation in the profession and overcome stereotypical notions about women's capacities in holding higher positions within medicine (i.e., the deficiency focus described in Chapter 2). The latter strategy is the route proposed by those who hold to the socialization theory and also those who represent the equal-opportunity perspective embraced by the liberal feminists.

There is another strand of this argument that clings to a more essentialist argument. The basis for the strategy would be an assets argument: women have special female skills and values that make them particularly apt to understand and to serve as advocates not only for women's issues but for all health issues. As a presidential address in the *American Journal of Public Health* recently suggested: "Women bring a humanistic view that has at its core respect for the individual woman, man, and child. Women bring a view that quality of life is the ultimate measure of our success. The women's agenda is for all of humanity" (Rodriguez-Trias 1994:1382).

The identification and elimination of the male-dominated medical discourse and the gendered premises of work would seem to be the solution suggested by the social constructionists. The deconstruction of medicine and its inherent male values and structures would be targets of such an endeavor that could be pursued by women both outside and inside medicine. The task would not be one solely pursued by women physicians in their capacity as experts. Instead, it could be a strategy for a larger coalition of women in various health professions and laywomen who together would promote a public health agenda that would integrate a so-called strategic essentialist stance on women's health. Such a view resembles the Foucauldian notion of medical knowledge: There is no absolute medical truth or a universal "women's health" concept but alternative medical discourses and views on women's health that are situated in time and space.

As the Russian context has informed us, the existence of women physicians has hardly had an influence on women's health. The statistics on women's poor health and the high abortion rates are more telling about the material conditions of women in the Soviet and postcommunist era than indicators of the impact of women physicians' role in advancing women's health. The health of Russian women might be the ultimate lesson that one can learn from the potential of women physicians: The health of women is foremost a matter of women's economic, political, and social position in society rather than merely a product of the proportion of women in the medical profession.

# 9

## Conclusions

For many observers of women's position in the labor market, the careers of women in the traditional professions—medicine, law, and the clergy—have become tests of gender equality and opportunities available for a new generation of women. Women's growing proportion among practicing physicians and among the new entrants to medical school has been viewed as a sign of such equality. Some skeptics point to the skewed career profile of women: women are highly represented at the bottom of the hierarchy of medicine but still sparsely distributed in the higher ranks of academic and administrative medicine. The skeptics see such a distribution as an indication that the initially envisioned genuine integration of women into medicine has not come to pass. The optimists try, however, to console the skeptics with current statistics: women constitute almost or already a majority of the medical school students in most Western countries today. From these statistics, the optimists draw the conclusion that women will in the near future head most of the organizations and hold most of the top positions in the profession. This view is based on a notion that there is a lag in the representation of women at medicine's higher levels. The assumption is that as the new and large cohort of women advances in its career, it will be evenly distributed and soon even outnumber men in most areas and ranks of medicine.

The Scandinavian evidence, however, reveals that women have not moved smoothly to positions of authority at anything like the rate predicted by their numbers at the entry level. In 1950, the proportion of women among Finnish doctors was the same as the proportion in U.S. medicine now, fifty years later. However, there is a much higher proportion of women in academic medicine in the United States than in any of the Scandinavian countries. So the question to be addressed in this concluding chapter is: Are there any reasons to believe that conditions now are different from the past?

This book has examined women physicians' careers and feminist agendas in three social and political settings: the United States, Scandinavia, and Russia/Soviet Union. The purpose has partly been to provide a historical account of women's entry into and current status in the medical profession in three different contexts and in this way set the stage for a comparison of the similarities but also marked differences in women's medical careers. The purpose has also been to address some feminist and sociological questions about how women can change their own conditions and create a health care system responding to women's health needs.

The question guiding the research reported here is this: How do we explain the vastly different proportions of women doctors in U.S., Scandinavian, and Russian medicine? The argument presented is that the history of women in medicine provides a lens for the examination of the changes in medicine. The study of women physicians illuminates the major transformations of medicine as a social organization and as a profession. The central point has been that women's presence and agendas illuminate the major scientific, professional, and organizational transformations in medicine. These transformations have had gendered implications.

In this concluding chapter, the first section will summarize the major conclusions of the individual chapters, which gave a descriptive account of women's representation in medicine in three different social and political contexts. The second section will address two questions related to the usefulness of various theoretical perspectives on women physicians' careers and the kind of changes that women physicians have made. The third section will address the question: What contributions are women physicians likely to make in the future?

## MEDICAL CAREERS AND FEMINIST AGENDAS:
## THE TALE OF THREE CONTEXTS

The preceding chapters have presented three key sociological issues—the numbers, medical practice, and feminist agendas—of women in U.S., Scandinavian, and Russian medicine during the past hundred years. In international terms, U.S. and Russian women were pioneers: Women practiced medicine earlier and constituted a higher proportion of the physicians in these countries than in most of the European countries with a long tradition of medicine and an organized medical profession. Women gained access to medical education in the 1860s and 1870s in the United States and Russia, but then mainly through gender-segregated medical education. At the turn of the century, women constituted about 6 percent of medical practitioners in the United States and Russia, and they provided forceful images of women's liberation and equal rights, especially in higher education and in the professions. Women in Scandinavia were influenced by these images. The women pioneers in Scandinavian medicine entered coeducational medical schools in the latter part of the nineteenth century but constituted a mere handful in each of the Scandinavian countries at the turn of the century.

In this book's presentation of women in medicine, the organization of medicine has been viewed as related to two societal institutions: the economy and the gender system. The larger economic and political organization of society provides the base for how medical care is organized. When the first cohort of women entered medical schools and eventually ventured out as practitioners in the latter part of the nineteenth century, health care was organized as a cottage industry: physicians worked as independent entrepreneurs in solo, fee-for-service practice. During the first decades of the twentieth century, hospital medicine introduced a new division of labor and hierarchical structure in medicine, an organizational structure that became a new barrier for women physicians. Obstacles to access to residencies and to the more prestigious specialized areas of medicine became invisible stumbling blocks to women's integration and advancement.

Chapters 3, 4, and 5 described the structural changes in medicine, proceeding from a cottage industry of solo practitioners, to a factory mode of production within the framework of hospital medicine, to the current corporate form of health care in U.S. medicine, to the adoption of market-oriented strategies in the Scandinavian welfare states, and to the ambiguous anomaly of Russian medicine. As shown in Chapter 3, the current corporate structure of U.S. medicine is changing the profession to an occupational group of employees, a status comparable to the salaried status of the Scandinavian and Russian physicians.

The early entry of women into U.S. and Russian medicine meant a practice mainly restricted to women and children. In all three settings, women physicians became involved in the public health movement at the turn of the century and they acted as powerful promoters of maternal and children's health programs and health legislation. A simultaneous bifurcation of the education and profession of scientific medicine and public health into two different schools and professional groups in the United States in the 1920s left women physicians without a constituency of their own and with few avenues to entering hospital medicine. With the rise of hospital medicine and new medical specialties, U.S. women physicians encountered new barriers: they were excluded from most available residencies and internships.

Scandinavian women physicians' position was early hampered by hospital medicine's and academic medicine's being part of the public sector, from which women physicians were legally barred until the 1910s and 1920s. This sector was part of male-mainstream medicine and characterized by a rigid hierarchical structure. For Soviet medicine, and later Scandinavian medicine, health care has been a decommodified public service provided by a universal health service system or insurance. State-organized medicine in the Soviet Union reduced the professional power of medicine and paradoxically returned medical education in the 1930s to the kind of vocational training and the status of doctors that had characterized U.S. medicine during the pre-Flexnerian period. But it was not salaried status and loss of control over medical education that resulted in the "feminization" of the medical profession in the Soviet Union (by 1940 62 percent and by 1950 77 percent of Soviet doctors were women). As shown in Chapter 5, growth of industrial production became the primary goal of the state-directed Soviet economic policy and jobs in the service sector were of secondary importance. Physicians were but one occupational group among other medical workers, and their salaries were considerably lower than the highest offered to (male)workers in industrial production.

The development of a public primary care system in Scandinavia during the past three decades has been a welfare-state initiative to promote equity in health care and to include health as a welfare-state goal. This changed the character of the physicians involved in that part of the public sector: Primary-care physicians became one of the welfare-state occupations serving the goals of the welfare state. This position as a welfare-state occupation has had two consequences for the medical profession: it entailed a sheltered labor market but it has also resulted in limited professional autonomy.

First, the primary care system became a new opportunity structure for young physicians in Scandinavia, a majority of whom since the 1990s have been women. This was a new practice setting that women physicians could gain control over—with, for example, fixed salary levels, set hours of work, and choice of part-time work. The public primary-care sector has offered women physicians in the Scandinavian context what Connell (1987:281) has called a "liberated zone": a physical and social space providing a relatively ungendered and nonhierarchical work environment.

Second, the Scandinavian public primary care system does not allow its practitioners the traditional professional autonomy enjoyed by solo, fee-for-service practitioners. U.S. observers have interpreted the trend toward salaried status as the ultimate sign of a trend toward a "proletarianization" and "feminization" of medicine. But it is not so much the salaried status and the influx of women as the changes in the fiscal structure that have influenced Scandinavian and Russian physicians' professional status during the past decade. The Scandinavian and the Russian health care systems have been characterized by a dominant public sector, but new decentralized ways of organizing and financing health care have emerged in these systems in the 1990s. The Scandinavian political system has increasingly transferred the political and economic responsibility for health care from the state to local government. Recent decentralization of financing and decision-making in health care in Sweden and Finland has meant that certain rationalizations have been introduced in local health care. The post-

World-War-II era of a homogeneous welfare-state national health service system ended in these two countries in the early 1990s. Instead, local governments—in concrete terms, local politicians—are the decision-makers about the kind of health care services provided by public or private agencies, even though both are still mainly financed by the public sector. The financial constraints have so far not resulted in major cuts in services but a more stringent budget for recruiting and financing health professionals, including physicians. Stress, overwork, and job insecurity have plagued the work conditions of Scandinavian physicians lately, because of unemployment and temporary appointments among them. Norway has here been an exception since a shortage of health professionals, including physicians, has characterized its health care delivery system.

In this book three approaches for interpreting women's position in medicine have been presented (Halford et al. 1997). First, the contingent approach suggests that organizations are fundamentally gender-neutral and their gendered character is the contingent outcome of specific historic circumstances rather than an intrinsic feature of bureaucratic organizations. The proponents of this approach would point out that women constituted 7 percent of the physicians in the United States in 1970, and 23 percent in 1999. In 1999–2000, 46 percent of entrants to U.S. medical schools were women, as compared to 9 percent in 1970. The latter figures could be seen as indicators that the normative barriers to women's career in medicine have fallen. The figures for Finland—in 2000, 67 percent of physicians under thirty were women—would also suggest that young women are socialized to other educational goals and role expectations than in the past.

The increasing proportion of women in U.S. and Scandinavian medicine certainly points to the eradication of normative barriers. On the other hand, the clustering of women in specialties that confirm the traditional caring skills of women (e.g., pediatrics) challenges this explanation. Furthermore, the small numbers of women in academic medicine and administrative structures of health care have been interpreted as evidence of the continuing existence of gatekeeping mechanisms and a male-dominated power structure. As Chapters 3, 4, and 5 have shown, women comprised 27 percent of the medical school faculty in the United States in 1999, compared to 19 percent in Finland, 13 percent in Norway, 8 percent in Denmark, and 6 percent in Sweden in 1996. (The latest figures for the Soviet Union were from the 1970s, when 20 percent of the medical faculty were women.) These figures point to the existence of a glass ceiling, a metaphor suggesting that the "obstacles women face to promotion relative to men systematically increase as they move up the hierarchy" (Baxter and Wright 2000:275). Considering that the Scandinavian medical profession is almost gender-balanced, the glass ceiling effect seems to be stronger than in the United States. This observation is further supported by Baxter and Wright's (2000) cross-national study of the gender gap in managerial jobs in the United States, Australia, and Sweden. In Sweden, women appeared to be particularly disadvantaged relative to men in moving from lower- to middle-management levels. The interpretation offered seems to apply for medicine as well. In liberal democratic policies, the focus of women's struggle against gender inequality is equal rights, which has led to affirmative action policies to eradicate structural barriers and thereby to eliminate discrimination that affects individual choices and opportunities. In social democratic politics, like those in Scandinavia, the core issue is the satisfaction of basic needs and the universal access to concomitant services, which has led to policies directed toward the decommodified provision of services (child care, maternal care, day care for children) and labor laws (parental leave) (ibid.:299). The latter policies have predominantly addressed inequalities generated by class rather than by gender.

These policy issues and strategies for change were further illuminated in Chapter 8, which addressed the question whether women's challenge of medicine has had more of an effect when pursued from within or from outside medicine. The chapter also addressed the question whether the women's health movement represents a missing feminist movement in Scandinavia. In the United States, women's health advocacy and the policy of inclusion (e.g., in clinical trials) have been based on an equal-rights policy, a policy that currently is further backed by women's lobbying groups at the federal level. This is a kind of politics that resembles the policymaking that in the Scandinavian context has been called "state feminism." The latter Scandinavian political heritage has resulted in the integration of women's health needs into health care provisions based on the principle of universal and public access. Gender equity is a public ideology in Scandinavia, a circumstance that has resulted in women's general trust in the public sector and its protection of women's interests. This is a widely held notion among women in Sweden and Finland, who do not tend to organize outside the labor unions' or political parties' women's caucuses where they present their views on policies to be enacted in the public sector. The lack of a vibrant lay advocacy movement among women in Sweden, Finland, and Norway (Denmark was shown to be an exception) has been reflected in the relative absence of a discussion about alternatives and about the kind of services that would meet different women's health needs. The prevailing notion is that (gender-neutral) experts, working as agents of the welfare-state, protect women from being exploited by unprofessional or profit-oriented commercial interests by defining women's health needs and by setting up standardized services within the public sector. This approach is different from the recent effort among feminist women's health advocates within academic medicine in the United States. Chapter 8 showed how the new area of women's health has given women in U.S. medicine a new jurisdiction and knowledge claim for the advancement of a new specialty in women's health. This jurisdictional claim can legitimate the emergence of a new specialist within the existing structure of medicine—the women's health physician. The women's health physician serves as an advocate for women's health needs as well as an expert and feminist promoter of medical knowledge on women's health.

Second, the essentialist approach to gender proposes that a bureaucratic organization is inherently a masculine form of organizing work or, alternatively, that caring is a special type of female competence. Some have tended to perceive women as bearers of a potential humanistic and holistic approach to medicine that would head the rest of the profession toward a substantial change in the way that medicine is practiced. This view suggests that women in medicine can make a special contribution, because women's skills complement men's. Still others interpret signs of gender segregation in medicine in cultural terms: women have been socialized differently from men so they have a different perspective and "culture." Women voluntarily choose to practice medicine in a way that will not impinge on their tasks as women. Hence, their high proportion in pediatrics (e.g., 46 percent in the United States and 58 percent in Finland) could be seen as a sign of women's conscious choosing and of resisting the traditional view of professional work that has been tailored according to male-gendered criteria of commitment and calling to heroic medicine like surgery.

Third, the embedded approach suggests that an organization like medicine can best be understood as a socially situated practice, and the argument is that gender is embedded in any organization. The prevailing notion of gender rests on a binary conceptualization of gender: There are two gender categories—men and women. This conceptualization has also tended to give higher status to men and thereby create a gender system that has a built-in gender inequality (Lorber 2000b, Ridgeway 1991). The embedded approach can be used to illuminate the structural features of current gender segregation of medicine rather than merely to see the uneven distribution of men and women among specialties as the aggregated outcome of individual choices based on sex-role expectations. The embedded approach sees the male-gendered master status of the profession, the gender segregation of specialties, and men's and women's different styles of practicing medicine as products of gendered social practices. Men and women are "doing" both gender and medicine at the same time. For example, the small number of women in surgery has been explained by pointing to the masculine medical discourse of surgery and to surgery's male-gendered character. Both social practices tend to exclude women on the basis of their gender, because women do not have the more valued (male) gender status and the valued competence attached to the nominal characteristic of being a man. As shown in Chapter 6, recent cross-national research on surgeons indicates that a masculine culture is valorized in surgery, a specialty that in the United States and Scandinavia has about 10 percent women.

*Gendered competencies* are embodied and by means of *gender typing*, specialties or tasks within specialties come to be seen as appropriate either for men or for women physicians. Chapter 7 showed that women are not always the victims of gendered practices but also themselves are actively involved in the social construction of discourses legitimating their claim to the mastery of a special expertise and competence in a specialty. Chapter 7 illuminated how gendered practices are interpreted to work in pathology. *Gender casting* was presented as a discursive strategy whereby women's practice is restricted to domains that confirm their traditional caring skills—for example, diagnosing children's tissues. *Gender inclusion*, by contrast, is another discursive counterstrategy, one whereby women claim to be carriers of a special female competence that encompasses the craft skills of the pathologist: the visualization and handicraft needed for microscopy.

## WHAT CAN WE LEARN ABOUT WOMEN'S MEDICAL CAREERS AND FEMINIST AGENDAS BY STUDYING WOMEN PHYSICIANS IN THREE CONTEXTS?

The overview of the medical careers and feminist agendas of U.S., Scandinavian, and Russian women physicians presented in this book provides an opportunity to address three central feminist questions about how women can change their own conditions and create a health care system that responds to women's health needs.

The first question is: What theories best explain the data on women physicians' careers? A second, related question is: What strategies seem to have the best payoff for women's advancement in medicine? Chapter 2 presented an overview of the theories in the sociology of professions and organizational theories on gender and organizations. Theories in the sociology of professions were found to be gender-neutral or gender-blind or then to address gender in a tacit way. The focus in theories on professions is the specific character of professions that defines them as different from other occupational groups. Such theories explain the specific power of professions and, from a feminist point of view, why professions historically have been male-dominated. These theories provide few analytical tools for explaining women's position in the profession. Socialization- and sex-role theories have, sociologically viewed, a limited explanatory power because they ultimately reduce the gender inequality in women's location horizontally and vertically in medicine to the result of the aggregate sum of individual choices.

By contrast, recent theory building in organizational theory has explicitly addressed women's position in organizations, mainly in large corporations. Most of these theories have been used to illuminate women's location at different levels of management. Since medicine is a hierarchical organization, these theories are useful in interpreting the cross-national data on women physicians. The glass-ceiling metaphor has the advantage of making the male-dominated and gendered power structure of organizations visible and pointing to the cumulative barriers that women are exposed to as they seek to advance in their career in medicine. This perspective provides a forceful image for policies that emphasize equal rights, gender equality, and special programs for women (affirmative action, women's support groups within a specialty, and women mentors for women in academe) that aim to eradicate structural barriers for women's career advancement.

The disadvantage with both socialization and gatekeeping theories is that they leave the underlying organizational structure and gender-based content of an organization intact.

The advantage of the embedded approach is that it addresses the gendered power of the organization of medicine and of the profession. It points to the hidden consensual cultural beliefs of gender as a nominal characteristic and the status value attached to male gender (Ridgeway 1991). In much of the work in medicine, competence is embodied in the form of a male physician. Gendered competence can be challenged by women if the gendered medical discourse and the gendered social practice confirming the division of labor are made visible. As indicated in this book, a totally ungendered practice of medicine might be an illusive goal, whereas a less gendered (female or male) practice of medicine seems a more realistic future.

## WHAT KIND OF IMPACT WILL WOMEN PHYSICIANS HAVE?

The third question is: What kind of changes have women physicians made and what contributions are women physicians likely to make in the future?[1] Several scholars in the field have resorted to Reskin and Roos's (1990) typology—genuine integration, ghettoization, or resegregation—when they have evaluated the future direction of gender and medicine (Riska and Wegar 1993b; Brooks 1998; Gjerberg 2001a) and made predictions about women's contributions to medicine. According to such a scheme, the prophecy of the ghettoization of U.S. women physicians into selected specialties, the gender-balanced character of the Scandinavian medical professions, and the resegregation of the Russian medical profession into men's work as the profession might regain its traditional status also serves as a gradient of women's potential contributions to medicine. Such an interpretation conflates the sex composition and the gender type of a profession and draws conclusions about the power over and impact on practice of one of the genders on the basis of its numerical representation (e.g., Britton 2000:424). Women's increasing numerical representation is certainly not an insignificant indicator of their influence in medicine. Women physicians have acted in the past, as they do currently, as powerful role models for working women, by challenging gender-typical notions about women's capacities in medicine. They have also historically and currently drawn attention to preventive and psychosocial aspects of medicine and been more alert than men physicians to certain underdiagnosed and over- or undertreated diseases among women (see Chapter 6). In such a capacity, women physicians will continue to change practice and to promote new medical knowledge about women's health.

Women's numerical representation should, however, not be confounded with the gendered character of medicine and its specialties. It is in this domain that women physicians, or any woman, can and should challenge medicine. Although evidence-based medicine in the area of women's health can be seen as a revival of "feminist empiricism" of the 1980s, it could for women physicians and women's health advocates be a heuristic device to identify and challenge the male-gendered practices of medicine. In doing medical research on women's and men's health from a gender perspective and in their own practice, women physicians can affect the content of medicine and the care of their patients.

The question raised in the beginning of the chapter is whether women will move up to positions of authority at the rate their number at entry level predicts. A related question is what impact, if any, they will have on the practice and on the content of medicine—e.g., through developing curricula from a gender-sensitive point of view. These questions might be answered in different ways by taking a contingent (gender-neutral), an essentialist, or an embedded approach.

According to a gender-neutral view, the prevailing notions of gender equality as a societal goal will move women to positions of authority faster than before, or at a rate commensurate with their gender-balanced or even numerical domination at entry level in the profession. But this viewpoint does not acknowledge that women in particular would bring anything new to the curriculum since they are by definition similar to men.

If answered in an essentialist way, the question would be rephrased as: Do women doctors want to perpetuate the existing medical hierarchy and the narrow biomedical view of medicine? There are certainly many women physicians who will like—if provided the opportunity—to moderate hierarchies by establishing women-friendly practices in primary care settings or in hospitals, which would reduce the social distance between patient and practitioner.

The embedded approach would not yield a universal answer to the foregoing questions but would suggest that the answer to both questions depends on how medicine is organized in the future.

The cross-national examination of women's careers presented in this book lends support to the argument that affirmative action programs are needed if women are to advance to positions of authority—as professors of medicine, as department heads of administrative and academic medicine—at an improved rate. But for the remaining women physicians, who work in the lower echelons of medicine, the question remains as to how they as insiders can change medicine. Obviously it will be hard for them to have any major impact unless they are supported by women in positions of authority inside or outside medicine and work in a health care system acknowledging the specific interests and values women are assumed to represent in medicine. There will still be other women who wish to promote a holistic approach to health and who will therefore adopt alternative therapies and choose to work outside medicine. Alternative medicine is an expanding field in the United States, Scandinavia, and, particularly, in Russia. The conclusion reached here is nevertheless that continuing support of women in regular medicine would be a better strategy for advancing women's careers and women's health needs and at the same time honoring the history of all those women physicians who over the past one hundred years have worked for the improvement of health.

Research on women physicians has in the past challenged many assumptions about gender in the major theories in the sociology of professions. So has this study. As health care systems and gender systems vary, so do the work conditions and status of both women physicians and of the field falling under the general rubric of "women's health." Both issues—women physicians and women's health—have been and will continue to be subject to women's movements, women's professional projects, and knowledge claims.

## NOTE

1. I am greatly indebted to Judith Lorber for pointing out this crucial question and for commenting on my answers to it.

# References

Abbott, Andrew. 1988. *The System of Professions: An Essay on the Division of Expert Labor*. Chicago: University of Chicago Press.

Acker, Joan. 1990. "Hierarchies, Jobs, Bodies: A Theory of Gendered Organizations." *Gender and Society* 4:139–58.

Acker, Joan. 1992. "Gendered Institutions: From Sex Roles to Gendered Institutions." *Contemporary Sociology* 21:565–69.

Alcoff, Linda. 1988. "Cultural Feminism Versus Post-Structuralism: The Identity Crisis in Feminist Theory." *Signs* 13:405–36.

Alessio, John C. and Julie Andrzejewski. 2000. "Unveiling the Hidden Glass Ceiling: An Analysis of the Cohort Effect Claim." *American Sociological Review* 65:311–15.

Altekruse, Joan M. and Susanne W. McDermott. 1987. "Contemporary Concerns of Women in Medicine." Pp. 65–88 in *Feminism within Science and Health Professions: Overcoming Resistance*, edited by S. V. Rossner. Oxford: Pergamon.

Alvesson, Mats and Yvonne Due Billing. 1997. *Understanding Gender and Organizations*. London: Sage.

American Medical Association. 2000. Website: www.ama-assn.org.

American Medical Women's Association. 2000. *AMWA Connections* 21(1).

Andersen, Margaret L. 1983. *Thinking About Women: Sociological and Feminist Perspectives*. New York: Macmillan.

Andersen, M. Robyn and Nicole Urban. 1997. "Physician Gender and Screening: Do Patient Differences Account for Differences in Mammography Use?" *Women and Health* 26:29–39.

Andreen, Andrea. [1956] 1988. *Karolina Widerström: En levnadsteckning*. Stockholm: Norstedts.

Apple, Rima D. (Ed.). 1990. *Women, Health, and Medicine in America: A Historical Handbook*. New York: Garland.

Armstrong, David. 1983. *The Political Anatomy of the Body: Medical Knowledge in Britain in the Twentieth Century*. Cambridge: Cambridge University Press.

Armstrong, David. 1995. "The Rise of Surveillance Medicine." *Sociology of Health and Illness* 17:393–404.

Armstrong, David. 1997. "Foucault and the Sociology of Health and Illness: A Prismatic Reading." Pp. 15–30 in *Foucault: Health and Medicine*, edited by Alan Petersen and Robin Bunton. London: Routledge.

Arnetz, Bengt B. 2001. "Psychosocial Challenges Facing Physicians of Today." *Social Science and Medicine* 52:203–13.

Association of American Medical Colleges. 1996. AAMC Paper: AAMC Project Committee on Increasing Women's Leadership in Academic Medicine. *Academic Medicine* 71:799–811.

Atkinson, J. Maxwell and Heritage, John (eds.). 1984. *Structures of Social Action: Studies of Conversation Analysis*. Cambridge: Cambridge University Press.

Atkinson, Paul. 1995. *Medical Talk and Medical Work: The Liturgy of the Clinic*. Thousand Oaks, CA: Sage.

Auerbach, Judith D. and Anne E. Figert. 1995. "Women's Health Research: Public Policy and Sociology." *Journal of Health and Social Behavior* (Extra issue):115–31.

Baker, Laurence C. 1996. "Differences in Earnings Between Male and Female Physicians." *The New England Journal of Medicine* 334:960–64.

Barnett, Rosalind C., Phyllis Carr, Alicia Dobashian Boisnier, Arlene Ash, Robert H. Friedman, Mark A. Moskowitz, and Laura Szalacha. 1998. "Relationships of Gender and Career Motivation to Medical Faculty Members' Production of Academic Publications." *Academic Medicine* 73:180–86.

Barr, Donald A. 1995. "The Professional Structure of Soviet Medical Care: The Relationship between Personal Characteristics, Medical Education and Occupational Setting for Estonian Physicians." *American Journal of Public Health* 85:373–78.

Barr, Donald A. and Mark G. Field. 1996. "The Current State of Health Care in the Former Soviet Union: Implications for Health Care Policy and Reform." *American Journal of Public Health* 86:307–12.

Barr, Donald A. and Rudi Schmid. 1996. "Medical Education in the Former Soviet Union." *Academic Medicine* 71:141–45.

Bart, Pauline B. 1987. "Seizing the Means of Reproduction: An Illegal Feminist Abortion Collective—How and Why It Worked." *Qualitative Sociology* 14: 339–57.

Barzansky, Barbara, Harry S. Jonas, and Sylvia I. Etzel. 2000. "Educational Programs in U.S. Medical Schools, 1999–2000." *Journal of the American Medical Association* 284:1114–20.

Baxter, Janeen and Erik Olin Wright. 2000. "The Glass Ceiling Hypothesis: A Comparative Study of the United States, Sweden, and Australia." *Gender and Society* 14:275–94.

Becker, Howard. S., Blanche Geer, Everett C. Hughes, and Anselm L. Strauss. 1961. *Boys in White: Student Culture in Medical School*. Chicago: University of Chicago Press.

Bensing, Jozien, Atie van den Brink-Muinen, and Dinny de Bakker. 1993. "Gender Differences in Practice Style: A Dutch Study of General Practice." *Medical Care* 31:221–29.

Bergstrand, Hilding. 1963. "Läkarekåren och provinsialläkareväsendet." Pp. 107–57 in *Medicinalväsendet i Sverige 1813–1962*, edited by Wolfram Kock. Stockholm: AB Nordiska Bokhandelns Förlag.

Berliner, Howard. 1975. "A Larger Perspective on the Flexner Report." *International Journal of Health Services* 5:573–92.

Berliner, Howard. 1982. "Medical Modes of Production." Pp. 162–73 in *The Problem of Medical Knowledge: Examining the Social Construction of Medicine*, edited by P. Wright and A. Treacher. Edinburgh: Edinburgh University Press.

Berliner, Howard. 1986. *A System of Scientific Medicine: Philanthropic Foundations in the Flexner Era*. New York: Routledge & Kegan Paul.

Bertakis, Klea D., L. Jay Helms, Edward J. Callahan, Rahman Azari, and John A. Robbins. 1995. "The Influence of Gender on Physician Practice Style." *Medical Care* 33:407–16.

Bickel, Janet. 2000. "Women in Academic Medicine." *Journal of the American Medical Women's Association* 55:10–12.

Billing, Yvonne Due. 1997. "Är ledarskap manligt, kvinnligt eller något annat." In *Ledare, makt och kön*, edited by Anita Nyberg and Elizabeth Sundin. Rapport till

Utredningen om fördelningen av ekonomisk makt och ekonomiska resurser mellan kvinnor och män. Stockholm: SOU 135.

Billing, Yvonne Due and Mats Alvesson. 1989. "Four Ways of Looking at Women and Leadership." *Scandinavian Journal of Management* 5:63–80.

Billings, Frank. 1923. "The Resourceful General Practitioner of Modern Medicine." *Journal of the American Medical Association* 80:519–24.

Blom, Ida. 1987. "Hjernen kan ikke udvikle sig samtidig med ovarierne . . . Kvinnelige leger; leger og kvinner i Norge omkring arhundreskiftet." Pp. 7–32 in *Kvinnliga forskarpionjärer i Norden*. Stockholm: JÄMFO, Rapport no. 8.

Blom, Ida. 1995. "'. . . Uden dog at overskride sin naturlige Begrænsning'—kvinner i Akademia, 1882–1932." Pp. 19–32 in *Alma Maters døtre: Et århundre med kvinner i akademisk utdanning*, edited by Suzanne Stiver Lie and Maj Birgit Rørslett. Oslo: Pax Forlag.

Blum, Linda and Vicki Smith. 1988. "Women's Mobility in the Corporation: A Critique of the Politics of Optimism." *Signs* 13:528–45.

Bonner, Thomas Neville. 1988. "Medical Women Abroad: A New Dimension of Women's Push for Opportunity in Medicine, 1850–1914." *Bulletin of the History of Medicine* 62:58–73.

Bonner, Thomas Neville. 1989. "Rendezvous in Zurich: Seven Who Made a Revolution in Women's Medical Education, 1864–1874." *Journal of the History of Medicine and Allied Sciences* 44:7–27.

Bordo, Susan R. 1993. *Unbearable Weight: Feminism, Western Culture and the Body*. Berkeley: University of California Press.

Boston Women's Health Book Collective. 1973. *Our Bodies, Ourselves: A Book by and for Women*. New York: Simon and Schuster.

Brandt, Allan M. and Martha Gardner. 2000. "Antagonism and Accommodation: Interpreting the Relationship between Public Health and Medicine in the United States during the 20th Century." *American Journal of Public Health* 90:707–15.

Bright, Cedric M., Corey A. Duefield, and Valerie E. Stone. 1998. "Perceived Barriers and Biases in the Medical Education Experience by Gender and Race." *Journal of the National Medical Association* 90:681–88.

Britt, Helena, Alice Bhasale, David A. Miles, Angelli Meza, Geoffrey P. Sayer, and Maria Angelis. 1996. "The Sex of the General Practitioner: A Comparison of Characteristics, Patients, and Medical Conditions Managed." *Medical Care* 34:403–15.

Britton, Dana M. 2000. "The Epistemology of the Gendered Organization." *Gender and Society* 14:418–34.

Brooks, Fiona. 1998. "Women in General Practice: Responding to the Sexual Division of Labour." *Social Science and Medicine* 47:181–93.

Broom, Dorothy H. 1991. *Damned If We Do: Contradictions in Women's Health Care*. Sydney: Allen & Unwin.

Broom, Dorothy H. and Roslyn V. Woodward. 1996. "Medicalization Considered: Toward a Collaborative Approach to Care." *Sociology of Health and Illness* 18:357–78.

Burger, Edward J., Mark G. Field, and Judyth L. Twigg. 1998. "From Assurance to Insurance in Russian Health Care: The Problematic Transition." *American Journal of Public Health* 88:755–58.

Buring, Julie E. 2000. "Women in Clinical Trials—A Portfolio for Success" (editorial). *New England Journal of Medicine* 343:505–6.

Burke, Ronald J. 1996. "Stress, Satisfaction and Militancy among Canadian Physicians: A Longitudinal Investigation." *Social Science and Medicine* 43:517–24.

Butler, Judith. 1993. *Bodies That Matter: On the Discursive Limits of Sex*. London: Routledge.

Carmel, Sara and Seymour M. Glick. 1996. "Compassionate-Empathic Physicians: Personality Traits and Social-Organizational Factors That Enhance or Inhibit this Behavior Pattern." *Social Science and Medicine* 43:1253–61.

Carpenter, Euginia S. 1977. "Women in Male-Dominated Health Professions." *International Journal of Health Services* 7:191–207.

Carpenter, Mick. 1993. "The Subordination of Nurses in Health Care: Towards a Social Divisions Approach." Pp. 95–130 in *Gender, Work and Medicine: Women and the Medical Division of Labour*, edited by Elianne Riska and Katarina Wegar. London: Sage.

Case, Susan M., Rose Hatala, Jennifer Blake, and Gerald S. Golden. 1999. "Does Sex Make a Difference? Sometimes It Does and Sometimes It Doesn't." *Academic Medicine* 74:37–40.

Cassell, Joan. 2000. *The Woman in the Surgeon's Body*. Cambridge, MA: Harvard University Press.

Chambers, Ruth and Jan Campbell. 1996. "Gender Differences in General Practitioners at Work." *British Journal of General Practice* 46:291–93.

Chapin Henry Dwight. 1921. "The Relation between the Child and Hospital Social Service." *Journal of the American Medical Association* 77:279–81.

Chavkin, Wendy. 1997. "Topics for Our Times: Affirmative Action and Women's Health" (editorial) *American Journal of Public Health* 87:732–34.

Chekhov, Anton. 1974. *Letters of Anton Chekhov*, edited by Avrahm Yarmolinsky. London: Jonathan Cape.

Chenet, Laurent. 2000. "Gender and Socio-Economic Inequalities in Mortality in Central and Eastern Europe." Pp. 182–207 in *Gender Inequalities in Health*, edited by Ellen Annandale and Kate Hunt. Buckingham: Open University Press.

Coburn, David. 1992. "Freidson Then and Now: An 'Internalist' Critique of Freidson's Past and Present Views of the Medical Profession." *International Journal of Health Services* 22:492–512.

Coburn, David. 1999. "Professions in Transition: Globalisation, Neo-Liberalism and the Decline of Medical Power." Pp. 139–56 in *Professional Identities in Transition: Cross-Cultural Dimensions*, edited by Inga Hellberg, Mike Saks, and Cecilia Benoit. Södertälje: Almqvist & Wiksell.

Cockerham, William C. 1997. "The Social Determinants of the Decline of Life Expectancy in Russia and Eastern Europe: A Lifestyle Explanation." *Journal of Health and Social Behavior* 38:117–30.

Cockerham, William C. 1999. *Health and Social Change in Russia and Eastern Europe*. London: Routledge.

Cohen, Jordan J. 1999. "Still Seeking Gender Equity in Health Care." *Academic Medicine* 74:1226.

Conley, Frances K. 1998. *Walking out on the Boys*. New York: Farrar, Straus and Giroux.

Connell, R. W. 1987. *Gender and Power: Society, the Person, and Sexual Politics*. Stanford, CA: Stanford University Press.

Conrad, Peter. 1992. "Medicalization and Social Control." *Annual Review of Sociology* 18:209–32.

Conrad, Peter. 2000. "Medicalization, Genetics, and Human Problems." Pp. 322–33 in *Handbook of Medical Sociology* (5th ed.), edited by Cloe E. Bird, Peter Conrad, and Alen M. Fremont. Upper Saddle River, NJ: Prentice Hall.

Cousins, O., A. Fugh-Berman, A. Kasper, C. Pearson, S. Ruzek, B. Seaman, N. Swenson, and A. Taylor. 1994. "The Women's Health Movement and Women Physicians" (letter to the editor). *Journal of Women's Health* 3:409–10.

Crawford, Robert. 1980. "Healthism and the Medicalization of Everyday Life." *International Journal of Health Services* 10:365–88.

Crawford, Robert. 1984. "A Cultural Account of 'Health': Control, Release, and the Social Body." Pp. 60–103 in *Issues in the Political Economy of Health Care*, edited by John B. McKinlay. New York: Tavistock.

Crompton, Rosemary, Nicky Le Feuvre, and Gunn Elisabeth Birkelund. 1999. "The Restructuring of Gender Relations within the Medical Profession." Pp. 179–200 in *Restructuring of Gender Relations and Employment*, edited by Rosemary Crompton. Oxford: Oxford University Press.

Curtis, Sarah, Natasha Petukhova, Galina Sezonova, and Nadia Netsenko. 1997. "Caught in the 'Traps of Managed Competition'? Examples of Russian Health Care Reforms from St. Petersburg and the Leningrad Region." *International Journal of Health Services* 27:661–86.

Dahle, Rannveig. 1994. "Women Doctors and Gendered Processes: The Case of Norway." In *Report of the 2nd European Feminist Research Conference 1994*, Graz, Austria.

Dahlerup, Drude. 1994. "Learning to Live with the State: State, Market, and Civil Society: Women's Need for State Intervention in East and West." *Women's Studies International Forum* 17:117–27.

Dahlerup, Drude. 1998. *Rødstrømperne: Den danske Rødstrømpebevægelses udvikling, nytænkning og gennemslag 1970–1985*. Parts 1 & 2. Copenhagen: Gyldendal.

Davies, Celia. 1996. "The Sociology of Professions and the Professions of Gender." *Sociology* 30:661–78.

Davis, Christopher M. 1990. "Economics of Soviet Public Health, 1928–1932." Pp. 146–72 in *Health and Society in Revolutionary Russia*, edited by Susan Gross Solomon and John F. Hutchinson. Bloomington: Indiana University Press.

Davis, Kathy. 1995. *Reshaping the Female Body: The Dilemma of Cosmetic Surgery*. London: Routledge.

De Koninck, Maria, Pierre Bergeron, and Renee Bourbonnais. 1997. "Women Physicians in Quebec." *Social Science and Medicine* 44:1825–32.

Dickie, Walter M. 1923. "The Place of Medicine in Public Health." *Journal of the American Medical Association* 81:1247–49.

Dodson, John M. 1923. "Preventive Medicine and the General Practitioner." *Journal of the American Medical Association* 80:1–6.

Doyal, Lesley. 1983. "Women, Health and the Sexual Division of Labor: A Case Study of the Women's Health Movement in Britain." *International Journal of Health Services* 13:373–87.

Drachman, Virginia G. 1984. *Hospital with a Heart: Women Doctors and the Paradox of Separatism at the New England Hospital, 1862–1969*. Ithaca, NY: Cornell University Press.

Drachman, Virginia G. 1986. "The Limits of Progress: The Professional Lives of Women Doctors, 1881–1926." *Bulletin of the History of Medicine* 60:58–72.

Dulmen, van A. M. and J. M. Bensing. 2000. "Gender Differences in Gynecologist Communication." *Women and Health* 30:49–61.

Edmondson, Linda H. 1984. *Feminism in Russia, 1900–1917*. London: Heinemann Educational Books.

Ehrenreich, Barbara and Deirdre English. 1973. *Witches, Midwives and Nurses: A History of Women Healers*. Old Westbury, NY: Feminist Press.

Ehrenreich, Barbara and Deirdre English. 1978. *For Her Own Good: 150 Years of the Experts' Advice to Women.* Garden City, NY: Anchor.

Einarsdottir, Gerda. 1999. "The Gendering of Status and Status of Gender: The Case of the Swedish Medical Profession." Pp. 175–94 in *Professional Identities in Transition: Cross-Cultural Dimensions,* edited by Inga Hellberg, Mike Saks, and Cecilia Benoit. Södertälje: Almqvist & Wiksell International.

Einarsdottir, Torgerdur. 1997. *Läkaryrket i förändring: En studie av den medicinska professionens heterogenisering och könsdifferentiering.* Ph.D. thesis. Department of Sociology, monograph no. 63, University of Gothenburg.

Elling, Ray. 1963. "The Hospital-Support Game in Urban Center." Pp. 73–111 in *The Hospital in Modern Society,* edited by Eliot Freidson. New York: Free Press.

Elstad, Jon Ivar. 1994. "Women's Priorities Regarding Physician Behavior and their Preference for a Female Physician." *Women and Health* 21:1–19.

Elzinga, Aant. 1990. "The Knowledge Aspect of Professionalization: The Case of Science-Based Nursing Education in Sweden." Pp. 151–73 in *The Formation of Professions: Knowledge, State and Strategy,* edited by R. Torstendahl and M. Burrage. London: Sage.

Engel, Barbara Alpern. 1979. "Women Medical Students in Russia, 1872–1882: Reformers or Rebels?" *Journal of Social History* 12:394–414.

Engman, Marja. 1987. "Många vägar till forskningen—kvinnliga forskarpionjärer i Finland." Pp. 33–60 in *Kvinnliga forskarpionjärer i Norden.* Rapport no. 8. Stockholm: JÄMFO.

Engman, Marja. 1996. *Det främmande ögat: Alma Söderhjelm i vetenskapen och offentligheten.* Helsingfors: Svenska litteratursällskapet i Finland.

Epstein, Cynthia Fuchs. 1970. *Woman's Place: Options and Limits in Professional Careers.* Berkeley: University of California Press.

Esping-Andersen, Gøsta. 1996. "After the Golden Age? Welfare State Dilemmas in a Global Economy." Pp. 1–31 in *Welfare States in Transition: National Adaptations in Global Economies,* edited by Gøsta Esping-Andersen, London: Sage.

Evans, Judith. 1995. *Feminist Theory Today: An Introduction to Second-Wave Feminism.* London: Sage.

Evertsson, Lars. 2000. "The Swedish Welfare State and the Emergence of Female Welfare State Occupations." *Gender, Work and Organization* 7:230–41.

Ewing, Sally. 1990. "The Science and Politics of Soviet Insurance." Pp. 69–96 in *Health and Society in Revolutionary Russia,* edited by Susan Gross Solomon and John F. Hutchinson. Bloomington: Indiana University Press.

Fang, Di, Ernest Moy, Lois Colburn, and Jeanne Hurley. 2000. "Racial and Ethnic Disparities in Faculty Promotion in Academic Medicine." *Journal of American Medical Association* 284:1085–92.

Farrell, Kathleen, Marlys Hearst Witte, Miguel Holguin, and Sue Lopez. 1979. "Women Physicians in Medical Academia: A National Statistical Survey." *Journal of American Medical Association* 241:2808–12.

Fee, Elizabeth. 1977. "Women and Health Care: A Comparison of Theories." Pp. 115–32 in *Health and Medical Care in the USA: A Critical Analysis,* edited by Vicente Navarro. Farmingdale, NY: Baywood.

Ferree, Myra Marx and Elaine J. Hall. 1996. "Rethinking Stratification from a Feminist Perspective: Gender, Race, and Class in Mainstream Textbooks." *American Sociological Review* 61:929–50.

Ferree, Myra Marx and Bandana Purkayastha. 2000. "Equality and Cumulative Disadvantage: Response to Baxter and Wright." *Gender and Society* 14:809–13.

Field, Mark. 1957. *Doctor and Patient in Soviet Russia.* Cambridge, MA: Harvard University Press.

Field, Mark. 1967. *Soviet Socialized Medicine: An Introduction*. New York: Free Press.
Field, Mark. 1975. "American and Soviet Medical Manpower: Growth and Evolution, 1910–1970." *International Journal of Health Services* 5:455–74.
Field, Mark. 1991. "The Hybrid Profession: Soviet Medicine." Pp. 43–62 in *Professions and the State: Expertise and Autonomy in the Soviet Union and Eastern Europe*, edited by Anthony Jones. Philadelphia: Temple University Press.
Field, Mark G. 2000. "The Health and Demographic Crisis in Post-Soviet Russia: A Two-Phase Development." Pp. 11–42 in *Russia's Torn Safety Nets: Health and Social Welfare During the Transition*, edited by Mark G. Field and Judyth L. Twigg. New York: St. Martin's.
Finnish Medical Association. 1990. *Physicians in Finland 1990*. (Leaflet)
Finnish Medical Association. 1996. *Lääkärikysely 1996: Tilastoja*. Helsinki: Tutkimusjaosto.
Finnish Medical Association. 2000. *Physicians in Finland 2000*. (Leaflet)
Finska Läkaresällskapet. 1875. Pp. 31–42 in Protokollen från Finska Läkaresällskapets allmänna möte i Helsingfors 28–29 maj 1873. Helsingfors: J. C. Frenkell & Son.
Finska Läkaresällskapet. 1900. Pp. 14–71 in Förhandlingar vid Finska Läkaresällskapets sjuttonde allmänna möte i Helsingfors den 21, 22, 23 september 1899. Helsingfors: Helsingfors centraltryckeri.
Fiorentine, Robert and Stephen Cole, 1992. "Why Fewer Women Become Physicians: Explaining the Premed Persistence Gap." *Sociological Forum* 7:469–96.
Firth-Cozens, Jenny. 2001. "Interventions to Improve Physicians' Well-Being and Patient Care." *Social Science and Medicine* 52:215–22.
Fisher, Sue. 1995. *Nursing Wounds: Nurse Practitioners, Doctors, Women Patients and the Negotiation of Meaning*. New Brunswick, NJ: Rutgers University Press.
Flexner, Abraham. 1910. "Medical Education in the United States and Canada. Basic Demographic and Professional Characteristics of US Women Physicians." *Bulletin of the Carnegie Foundation for the Advancement of Teaching*. No. 4.
Foucault, Michel. 1975. *The Birth of the Clinic*. New York: Vintage.
Fox, Nicolas J. 1992. *The Social Meaning of Surgery*. Milton Keynes: Open University Press.
Freedman, Estelle. 1979. "Separatism as Strategy: Female Institution Building and American Feminism, 1870–1930." *Feminist Studies* 5:512–29.
Freidson, Eliot. 1970. *Profession of Medicine*. New York: Mead.
Freidson, Eliot. 1984. "The Changing Nature of Professional Control." *Annual Review of Sociology* 10:1–20.
Freidson, Eliot. 1985. "The Reorganization of the Medical Profession." *Medical Care Review* 42:11–35.
Garpenby, Peter. 1989. *The State and the Medical Profession: A Cross-National Comparison of the Health-Policy Arena in the United Kingdom and Sweden 1945–1985*. Linköping University: Linköping.
Garpenby, Peter. 1999. "Resource Dependency, Doctors and the State: Quality Control in Sweden." *Social Science and Medicine* 49:405–24.
Geyer-Kordesch, Johanna. 1983. "Vorkämpferinnen im Ärzteberuf: Der Einstieg Angelsächsisher Frauen in Die professionalisierte Medizin des 19. Jahrhunderts." *Feministische Studien* 2:24–45.
Gjerberg, Elisabeth. 2001a. "Medical Women—Towards Full Integration? An Analysis of the Specialty Choices Made by Two Cohorts of Norwegian Doctors." *Social Science and Medicine* 52:331–43.
Gjerberg, Elisabeth. 2001b. "Gender Similarities in Doctors' Preferences—and Gender Differences in Final Specialisation." *Social Science and Medicine*. In Press.

Gjerberg, Elisabeth and Dag Hofoss. 1998. 'Dette er ikke noe for småjenter.' Legers forståelse av kjønnsforskjeller i spesialitetsvalg." *Tidsskrift for samfunnsforskning* 39:3–27.

Gjerberg, Elisabeth and Lise Kjølsrød. 2001. "The Doctor-Nurse Relationship: How Easy Is It to Be a Female Doctor Co-Operating with a Female Nurse?" *Social Science and Medicine* 52:189–202.

Glaser, Barney G. and Anselm L. Strauss. 1967. *The Discovery of Grounded Theory: Strategies for Qualitative Research*. Hawthorne, NY: Aldine de Gruyter.

Goffman, Erving. 1959. *The Presentation of Self in Everyday Life*. New York: Doubleday/Anchor.

Goffman, Erving. 1961. *Asylums*. Garden City, NY: Anchor.

Gray, Gwen. 1998. "How Australia Came to Have a National Women's Health Policy." *International Journal of Health Services* 28:107–25.

Gross, Edith B. 1992. "Gender Differences in Physician Stress." *Journal of the American Medical Women's Association* 47:107–112.

Gross, Edith B. 1997. "Gender Differences in Physician Stress: Why the Discrepant Findings?" *Women and Health* 26:1–14.

Haas, Jennifer. 1998. "The Cost of Being a Woman" (editorial). *New England Journal of Medicine* 338:1694–95.

Haavio-Mannila, Elina. 1975. *Sex Roles among Physicians and Dentists in Scandinavia*. Department of Sociology, research report No. 206, University of Helsinki.

Hafferty, Frederic W. 1988. "Cadaver Stories and the Emotional Socialization of Medical Students." *Journal of Health and Social Behavior* 29:344–56.

Hafferty, Frederic W. and John B. McKinlay. 1993. *The Changing Medical Profession: An International Perspective*. New York: Oxford University Press.

Halford, Susan, Mike Savage, and Anne Witz. 1997. *Gender, Careers and Organizations*. London: Macmillan.

Hall, Judith A., Julie T. Irish, Debra L. Roter, Carol M. Ehrlich, and Lucy H. Miller. 1994. "Satisfaction, Gender and Communication in Medical Visits." *Medical Care* 32:1216–31.

Harding, Sandra. 1991. *Whose Science? Whose Knowledge? Thinking from Women's Lives*. Ithaca, NY: Cornell University Press.

Hartsock, Nancy. 1983. "The Feminist Standpoint: Developing the Ground for a Specifically Feminist Historical Materialism." Pp. 283–310 in *Discovering Reality*, edited by Sandra Harding and Merill Hintikka. Dordrecht: Reidel.

Haug, Marie R. 1975. "The Deprofessionalization of Everyone?" *Sociological Focus* 8:197–213.

Haxthausen, Susie. 1993. *Historien om foreningen føreldre og fødsel*. København: DIKE.

Healy, Bernadine P. 1995. "Women's Health: The Third Suffrage Movement." *Journal of Women's Health* 4:219–20.

Hekman, Susan. 1997. "Truth and Method: Feminist Standpoint Theory Revisited." *Signs* 22:341–65.

Helmuth, Laura. 2000. "Reports See Progress, Problems in Trials." *Science* 288:1562–63.

Hinze, Susan W. 1999. "Gender and the Body of Medicine or at Least Some Body Parts: (Re)Constructing the Prestige Hierarchy of Medical Specialties." *Sociological Quarterly* 40:217–39.

Hinze, Susan W. 2000. "Inside Medical Marriages: The Effect of Gender on Income." *Work and Occupations* 27:464–99.

Hofoss, Dag, Sidney Flower, Jan Gertz, and Mauri Isokoski. 1983. *Helsepersonell i Norden, 1980–1990*. Report No. 7. Oslo: NAVSs Gruppe for Helsetjenesteforskning.

Hofstadter, Richard. 1955. *The Age of Reform.* New York: Vintage.

Holloway, Robert G., Jay Artis, and Walter Freeman. 1963. "The Participation Patterns of 'Economic Influentials' and the Control of a Hospital Board of Trustees." *Journal of Health and Human Behavior* 4:88–99.

Hovig, Berit. 1993. "Kvinner i medisinens akademi." *Tidsskrift for Den norske lægeforening* 113:2117–20.

Huber, Evelyne and John D. Stephens. 2000. "Partisan Governance, Women's Employment, and the Social Democratic Service State." *American Sociological Review* 65:323–42.

Hughes, Everett C. 1945. "Dilemmas and Contradictions of Status." *American Journal of Sociology* 50:353–59.

Hughes, Everett C. 1958. *Men and Their Work.* Glencoe, IL: Free Press.

Hutchinson, John F. 1990. " 'Who Killed Cock Robin?' An Inquiry into the Death of Zemstvo Medicine." Pp. 3–26 in *Health and Society in Revolutionary Russia,* edited by Susan Gross Solomon and John F. Hutchinson. Bloomington: Indiana University Press.

James, Jacquelyn B. 1997. "What Are the Social Issues Involved in Focusing on Difference in the Study of Gender?" *Journal of Social Issues* 53:213–32.

Johnson, Karen and Laurel Dawson. 1990. "Women's Health as a Multidisciplinary Specialty: An Exploratory Proposal." *Journal of the American Medical Women's Association* 45:222–24.

Johnson, Karen and Eileen Hoffman. 1993. "Women's Health: Designing and Implementing an Interdisciplinary Specialty." *Women's Health Issues* 3:115–19.

Johnson, Terry, Gerry Larkin, and Mike Saks, eds. 1995. *Health Professions and the State in Europe.* London: Routledge.

Jones, Anthony (Ed.). 1991. *Professions and the State: Expertise and Autonomy in the Soviet Union and Eastern Europe.* Philadelphia: Temple University Press.

Jørgensen, Line Holst. 1993. *Krop til tiden: en læsning af "Kvinde kend din krop."* Unpublished report. Copenhagen: Center for Women's Studies.

*Journal of the American Medical Association.* 1923. "Medical Education in the United States: Annual Presentation of Educational Data for 1923 by the Council on Medical Education and Hospitals." *Journal of the American Medical Association* 81:549–76.

*Journal of the American Medical Association.* 1930. "Proposed Resurrection of Sheppard-Townerism" (editorial). *Journal of the American Medical Association* 94:1240–41.

Kanter, Rosabeth Moss. 1977. *Men and Women of the Corporation.* New York: Basic Books.

Kassirer, Jerome P.. 1998. "Doctor Discontent" (editorial). *New England Journal of Medicine* 339:1543–44.

Katz, Pearl. 1999. *The Scalpel's Edge: The Culture of Surgeons.* Boston: Allyn & Bacon.

Katz-Rothman, Barbara. 1998. *Genetic Maps and Human Imaginations: The Limits of Science in Understanding Who We Are.* New York: W.W. Norton.

Kauppinen, Kaisa, Lyudmila Yasnaya, and Irja Kandolin. 1996. "Medical Doctors in Moscow: Their Work, Family and Well-Being." Pp. 164–74 in *Women's Voices in Russia Today,* edited by Anna Rotkirch and Elina Haavio-Mannila. Dartmouth: Aldershot.

Kauppinen-Toropainen, Kaisa. 1993. "Comparative Study of Women's Work Satisfaction and Work Commitment: Research Findings from Estonia, Moscow, and Scandinavia." Pp. 197–214 in *Democratic Reform and the Position of Women in Transitional Economies,* edited by Valentine M. Moghadam. Oxford: Clarendon.

Keller, Evelyn Fox 1983. *A Feeling for the Organism: The Life and Work of Barbara McClintock*. New York: W.H. Freeman.

Kimmel, Michael. 2000. "Saving the Males: The Sociological Implications of the Virginia Military Institute and the Citadel." *Gender and Society* 14:494–516.

Kirschstein, Ruth L. 1996. "Women Physicians: Good News and Bad News" (editorial). *The New England Journal of Medicine* 334:982–83.

Klawiter, Maren. 1999. "Racing for the Cure, Walking Women, and Toxic Touring: Mapping Cultures of Action within the Bay Area Terrain of Breast Cancer." *Social Problems* 46:104–26.

Kletke, Philip R., David W. Emmons, and Kurt D. Gillis. 1996. "Current Trends-Physicians' Practice Arrangements: From Owners to Employees." *Journal of the American Medical Association* 276:555–60.

Kletke, Philip R., William D. Marder, and Anne B. Silberger. 1990. "The Growing Proportion of Female Physicians: Implications for U.S. Physician Supply." *American Journal of Public Health* 80:300–4.

Koch, Lene. 1996. *Racehygiejne i Danmark, 1912–1956*. Copenhagen: Gyldendal.

Korremann, Grete. 1994. "Læger og køn—Spiller det en rolle?" *TemaNord* 1994:597 (Copenhagen: Nordic Council of Ministers).

Korvajärvi, Päivi. 1997. "Working within and between Hierarchies." Pp. 66–80 in *Gendered Practices in Working Life*, edited by Liisa Rantalaiho and Tuula Heiskanen. London: Macmillan.

Larson, Magali S. 1977. *The Rise of Professionalism*. Berkeley: University of California Press.

Le Feuvre, Nicky. 1999. "The Professional and Domestic Identities of Women Doctors in Britain and France." Pp. 195–213 in *Professional Identities in Transition: Cross-Cultural Dimensions*, edited by Inga Hellberg, Mike Saks, and Cecilia Benoit. Södertälje: Almqvist & Wiksell International.

Leonard, Julie C. and Kathleen E. Ellsbury. 1996. "Gender and Interest in Academic Careers among First- and Third-Year Residents." *Academic Medicine* 71:502–4.

Levinson, Daniel J. 1967. "Medical Education and the Theory of Adult Socialization." *Journal of Health and Social Behavior* 8:253–64.

Lindeman, Sari, Esa Läärä, Helinä Hakko, and Jouko Lönnqvist. 1996. "A Systematic Review on Gender-Specific Suicide Mortality in Medical Doctors." *British Journal of Psychiatry* 168:274–79.

Lindgren, Gerd. 1999. *Klass, kön och kirurgi: Relationer bland vårdpersonal i organisationsförändringarnas spår*. Malmö: Liber.

Long, Susan Orpett. 1986. "Roles, Careers and Femininity in Biomedicine: Women Physicians and Nurses in Japan." *Social Science and Medicine* 22:81–90.

Looker, Patty. 1993. "Women's Health Centers: History and Evolution." *Women's Health Issues* 3:95-100.

Lorber, Judith. 1975. "Women and Medical Sociology: Invisible Professionals and Ubiquitous Patients." Pp. 75–105 in *Another Voice: Feminist Perspective on Social Life and Social Science*, edited by Marcia Millman and Rosabeth Moss Kanter. New York: Anchor Press/Doubleday.

Lorber, Judith. 1984. *Women Physicians: Careers, Status, and Power*. London: Tavistock.

Lorber, Judith. 1985. "More Women Physicians: Will It Mean More Humane Health Care?" *Social Policy* 16(summer):50–54.

Lorber, Judith. 1993. "Why Women Physicians Will Never Be True Equals in the American Medical Profession." Pp. 62–76 in *Gender, Work and Medicine: Women and the Medical Division of Labour*, edited by Elianne Riska and Katarina Wegar. London: Sage.

Lorber, Judith. 1994. *Paradoxes of Gender*. New Haven, CT: Yale University Press.

Lorber, Judith. 1996. "Believing Is Seeing: Biology as Ideology." *Gender and Society* 7:568–81.

Lorber, Judith. 1997. *Gender and the Social Construction of Illness*. Thousand Oaks, CA: Sage.

Lorber, Judith. 1998. *Gender Inequality: Feminist Theories and Politics*. Los Angeles, CA: Roxbury.

Lorber, Judith. 2000a. "What Impact Have Women Physicians Had on Women's Health?" *Journal of the American Medical Women's Association* 55:13–15.

Lorber, Judith. 2000b. "Using Gender to Undo Gender: A Feminist Degendering Movement." *Feminist Theory* 1:79–95.

Löyttyniemi, Vappu. 2000. "'Töitä nuorille kollegoille'—Miten lääkärityöt-tömyyskeskustelussa rakennettiin lääkäriyttä." *Sosiaalilääketieteellinen Aika-kauslehti* 37:232–44.

Luksha, Olesya V. and Valery Mansurov. 1998. "Ways to Private Medicine in Modern Russia." Paper presented at the 16th World Congress of Sociology, Montreal, July 26–August 1

Lupton, Deborah. 1997. "Foucault and the Medicalization Critique." Pp. 94–110 in *Foucault: Health and Medicine*, edited by Alan Petersen and Robin Bunton. London: Routledge.

Lurie, Nicole, Jonathan Slater, Paul McGovern, Jacqueline Ekstrum, Lois Quam, and Karen Margolis. 1993. "Preventive Care for Women: Does the Sex of the Physician Matter?" *New England Journal of Medicine* 329:478–82.

Maheux, Brigitte, Francine Dufort, François Béland, André Jacques, and Anne Lévesque. 1990. "Female Practitioners: More Preventive and Patient Oriented?" *Medical Care* 28:87–92.

Marieskind, Helen. 1975. "The Women's Health Movement." *International Journal of Health Services* 5:217–23.

Marks, Geoffrey and William K. Beatty. 1972. *Women in White*. New York: Charles Scribner's Sons.

Marland, Hilary. 1995. "'Pioneer Work on All Sides': The First Generations of Women Physicians in the Netherlands, 1879–1930." *Journal of the History of Medicine and Allied Sciences* 50:441–77.

Martin, Emily. 1991. "The Egg and the Sperm: How Science Has Constructed a Romance Based on Stereotypical Male-Female Roles." *Signs* 16:485–501.

Martin, Steven C., Robert M. Arnold, and Ruth M. Parker. 1988. "Gender and Medical Socialization." *Journal of Health and Social Behavior* 29:333–43.

Mattila-Lindy, Sirpa, Elina Hemminki, Maili Malin, Katri Makkonen, Päivi Topo, Taina Mäntyranta, and Ilka Kangas. 1997. "Physicians' Gender and Clinical Opinions of Reproductive Health Matters." *Women and Health* 26: 15–26.

McCormick, Janice, Sheryl Reimer Kirkham, and Virginia Hayes. 1998. "Abstracting Women: Essentialism in Women's Health Research." *Health Care for Women International* 19:495–504.

McKinlay, John B. 1996. "Some Contributions from the Social System to Gender Inequalities in Heart Disease." *Journal of Health and Social Behavior* 37:1–26.

McKinlay, John B. and Joan Arches. 1985. "Towards the Proletarianization of Physicians." *International Journal of Health Services* 15:161–95.

McKinlay, John B. and Lisa D. Marceau. 1998. "The End of the Golden Age of Doctoring." Invited presentation at the annual meeting of the American Public Health Association, Washington, D.C., November.

McKinlay, John B. and John D. Stoeckle. 1988. "Corporatization and the Social Transformation of Doctoring." *International Journal of Health Services* 18:191–205.

McLean, John D. 1921. "Imperative Need of Union of the Medical Profession and the Health Authorities." *Journal of the American Medical Association* 77:827.

McMurray, Julia E., Mark Linzer, Thomas R. Konrad, et al. 2000. "The Work Lives of Women Physicians: Results from the Physician Work Life Study." *Journal of General Internal Medicine* 15:372–80.

Meeuwesen, Ludwien, Cas Schaap, and Cees van der Staak. 1991. "Verbal Analysis of Doctor-Patient Communication." *Social Science and Medicine* 32:1143–50.

Merton, Robert K, George Reader, and Patricia Kendall. 1957. *The Student Physician*. Cambridge, MA: Harvard University Press.

Mishler, Eliott G. 1984. *The Discourse of Medicine: Dialectics of Medical Interviews*. Norwood, NJ: Ablex.

Moldow, Gloria. 1987. *Women Doctors in Gilded-Age Washington: Race, Gender and Professionalization*. Urbana: University of Illinois Press.

Moran, Michael and Bruce Wood. 1993. *States, Regulation and the Medical Profession*. Buckingham: Open University Press.

Morantz, Regina Markell. 1977a. "Nineteenth-Century Health Reform and Women: A Program of Self-Help." Pp. 73–93 in *Medicine without Doctors: Home Health Care in American History*, edited by Guenther B. Risse, Ronald L. Numbers, and Judith Waltzer. New York: Science History Publications/Neale Watson Academic Publications.

Morantz, Regina Markell. 1977b. "Making Women Modern: Middle-Class Women and Health Reform in 19th Century America." *Journal of Social History* 4:490–507.

Morantz-Sanchez, Regina. 1985. *Sympathy and Science: Women Physicians in American Medicine*. New York: Oxford University Press.

Morantz-Sanchez, Regina. 1990. "Physicians." Pp. 477–95 in *Women, Health and Medicine in America: A Historical Handbook*, edited by Rima D. Apple. New York. Garland.

More, Ellen S. 1999. *Restoring the Balance: Women Physicians in the Profession of Medicine, 1850–1995*. Cambridge, MA: Harvard University Press.

Morgen, Sandra. 1986. "The Dynamics of Cooptation in a Feminist Health Clinic." *Social Science and Medicine* 23:201–10.

Moser, James W. 1998. "Physician Income Trends in the Last Ten Years." Pp. 29–37 in *Socioeconomic Characteristics of Medical Practice 1997/1998*, edited by Martin L. Gonzalez and Puling Zhang. Washington, DC: AMA, Center for Health Policy Research.

Nabel, Elizabeth G. 2000. "Coronary Heart Disease in Women—An Ounce of Prevention" (editorial.) *New England Journal of Medicine* 343:572–74.

Navarro, Vicente. 1975. "The Political Economy of Medical Care: An Explanation of the Composition, Nature, and Functions of the Present Health Sector of the United States." *International Journal of Health Services* 5:65–94.

Navarro, Vicente. 1976. *Medicine under Capitalism*. New York: Prodist.

Navarro, Vicente. 1977. *Social Security and Medicine in the USSR: A Marxist Critique*. Lexington, MA: Lexington.

Nettleton, Sarah. 1995. *The Sociology of Health and Illness*. Cambridge: Polity Press.

Nonnemaker, Lynn. 2000. "Women Physicians in American Medicine. New Insights from Cohort Studies." *New England Journal of Medicine* 342:399–405.

Nordic Medical Associations. 1996. *Den framtida läkararbetsmarknaden i Norden*. Stockholm: Norstedts tryckeri.

Nordic Medical Associations. 2000. *Physicians in the Nordic countries 2000* (leaflet). Stockholm: Author.

Nore, Anne Kathrine. 1993. "Fra nevenyttig jente til entusiastisk kirurg: En kvalitativ studie av kvinnelige kirurger i Norge." Spesialoppgave i helseadministrasjonsstudiet. Oslo: Universitetet i Oslo.

Norwegian Medical Association. 2000. *Legestatistikk 2000*. (Leaflet). Oslo.

Ohlander, Ann-Sofie. 1987. "Kvinnliga nordpolsfarare? De första kvinnliga forskarna i Sverige." Pp. 61–99 in *Kvinnliga forskarpionjärer i Norden* Stockholm: JÄMFO, report no. 8.

Oinas, Elina. 1998. "Medicalization by Whom: Accounts of Menstruation Conveyed by Young Women and Medical Experts in Medical Advisory Columns." *Sociology of Health and Illness* 20:52–70.

Parkin, Frank. 1979. *Marxism and Class Theory*. New York: Columbia University Press.

Parsons, Talcott. 1949. *Essays in Sociological Theory: Pure and Applied*. Glencoe, IL: Free Press.

Parsons, Talcott. 1951. *The Social System*. New York: Free Press.

Parsons, Talcott. 1979. "Definitions of Health and Illness in the Light of American Values and Social Structure." Pp. 120–44 in *Patients, Physicians and Illness* (3rd ed.), edited by E. Gartly Jaco. New York: Free Press.

Parvio, Salme. 1987. "Suomen naislääkärit 1900–1910." Pp. 18–20 in *Suomen Naislääkäri Yhdistys, r.y., Finlands Kvinnliga Läkares Förening r.f.* Helsinki: Kaivopuiston kirjapaino OY.

Pasko, Thomas and Bradley Seidman. 1999. *Physician Characteristics and Distribution in the U.S.: 1999 Edition*. Chicago: American Medical Association, Department of Data Survey and Planning.

Peräkylä, Anssi. 1995. *AIDS Counseling: Institutional Interaction and Clinical Practice*. Cambridge: Cambridge University Press.

Peräkylä, Anssi. 1997. "Conversational Analysis: A New Model of Research in Doctor-Patient Communication." *Journal of the Royal Society of Medicine* 90:205–8.

Perrow, Charles. 1963. "Goals and Power Structures: An Historical Case Study." Pp. 112–45 in *The Hospital in Modern Society*, edited by Eliot Freidson. New York: Free Press.

Petersson, Birgit. 1998. "Nielsine Nielsen: Förste kvindelige praktiserende læge." *Månadsskrift for praktiserende lægegern* 76:25–28.

Petersson, Birgit and Christen Sørensen. 1994. *Historien om en høring*. Copenhagen: Division of Social Medicine, University of Copenhagen.

Pfeffer, Jeffrey. 1973. "Size and Composition and Function of Hospital Boards of Directors: A Study of Organization Environment Linkages." *Administrative Science Quarterly* 18:349–64.

Pinn, Vivian W. 1999. "Women's Health Research: Progress and Future Directions." *Academic Medicine* 74:1104–5.

Porter, Sam. 1992. "Women in a Women's Job: The Gendered Experience of Nurses." *Sociology of Health and Illness* 14:510–27.

Pringle, Rosemary. 1998. *Sex and Medicine: Gender, Power, and Authority in the Medical Profession*. Cambridge: Cambridge University Press.

Psathas, George. 1995. *Conversation Analysis: The Study of Talk in Interaction*. London: Sage.

Ramer, Samuel C. 1990. "Feldshers and Rural Health Care in the Early Soviet Period." Pp. 121–45 in *Health and Society in Revolutionary Russia*, edited by Susan Gross Solomon and John F. Hutchinson. Bloomington: Indiana University Press.

Rantalaiho, Liisa. 1997. "Contextualising Gender." Pp. 16–30 in *Gendered Practices in Working Life*, edited by Liisa Rantalaiho and Tuula Heiskanen. London: Macmillan.

Rantalaiho, Liisa and Tuula Heiskanen. 1997. *Gendered Practices in Working Life*. London: Macmillan.

Rayan, Michael. 1989. *Doctors and the State in the Soviet Union*. London: Macmillan.

Rayan, Michael and Thomas Ray. 1996. "Trends in the Supply of Medical Personnel in the Russian Federation." *Journal of the American Medical Association* 276:339–42.

Relman, Arnold S. 1989. "The Changing Demography of the Medical Profession." *New England Journal of Medicine* 321:1540–41.

Reskin, Barbara F. and Debra Branch McBrier. 2000. "Why Not Ascription: Organisations' Employment of Male and Female Managers." *American Sociological Review* 65:210–33.

Reskin, Barbara F. and Patricia A. Roos. 1990. *Job Queues, Gender Queues: Explaining Women's Inroads into Male Occupations*. Philadelphia: Temple University Press.

Ridgeway, Cecilia. 1991. "The Social Construction of Status Value: Gender and Other Nominal Characteristics." *Social Forces* 70:367–86.

Riska, Elianne. 1993. "The Medical Profession in the Nordic Countries." Pp. 150–61 in *The Changing Medical Profession: An International Perspective*, edited by Frederic W. Hafferty and John B. McKinlay. New York: Oxford University Press.

Riska, Elianne. 1995. "They Don't Care: Unemployed Physicians in the Nordic Countries." *International Journal of Health Services* 25:259–69.

Riska, Elianne. 2001. "Towards Gender Balance: But Will Women Physicians Have an Impact on Medicine?" *Social Science and Medicine* 52:179–87.

Riska, Elianne and Katarina Wegar (Eds). 1993a. *Gender, Work and Medicine: Women and the Medical Division of Labour*. London: Sage.

Riska, Elianne and Katarina Wegar. 1993b. "Women Physicians: A New Force in Medicine?" Pp. 77–93 in *Gender, Work and Medicine: Women and the Medical Division of Labour*, edited by Elianne Riska and Katarina Wegar. London: Sage.

Riska, Elianne and Katarina Wegar. 1995. "The Medical Profession in the Nordic Countries: Medical Uncertainty and Gender-Based Work." Pp. 200–12 in *Health Professions and the State in Europe*, edited by Terry Johnson, Gerry Larkin, and Mike Saks. London: Routledge.

Roback, Gene, Diane Mead, and Lillian Randolph. 1986. *Physician Characteristics and Distribution in the U.S.* Chicago: American Medical Association.

Rodriguez-Trias, Helen. 1994. "Women Are Organizing: Environmental and Population Policies Will Never Be the Same" (1993 Presidential Address). *American Journal of Public Health* 84:1379–82.

Rogers, Naomi. 1990. "Women and Sectarian Medicine." Pp. 281–310 in *Women, Health, and Medicine in America: A Historical Handbook*, edited by Rima D. Apple. New York: Garland.

Rosenbeck, Bente. 1987. "Ud til grænserne—og lidt længere." Pp. 101–44 in *Kvinnliga forskarpionjärer i Norden*. Stockholm: JÄMFO, Report no. 8.

Rosser, Sue V. 1993. "A Model for a Specialty in Women's Health." *Journal of Women's Health* 2:99–104.
Roter, Debra L. and Judith A. Hall. 1998. "Why Physician Gender Matters in Shaping the Physician-Patient Relationship." *Journal of Women's Health* 7:1093–97.
Roter, Debra, M. Lipkin, and A. Korsgaard. 1991. "Sex Differences in Patients' and Physicians' Communication during Primary Care Visits." *Medical Care* 29:1083–93.
Roter, Debra L., Moira Stewart, Samuel M. Putnam, Mack Lipkin, William Stiles, and Thomas Inui. 1997. "Communication Patterns of Primary Care Physicians." *Journal of American Medical Association* 277:350–56.
Rothman, Sheila M. 1978. *Women's Proper Place: A History of Changing Ideals and Practices, 1870 to Present.* New York: Basic Books.
Rothstein, William. 1972. *American Physicians in the Nineteenth Century: From Sects to Science.* Baltimore, MD: Johns Hopkins University Press.
Ruzek, Sheryl Burt. 1978. *The Women's Health Movement: Feminist Alternatives to Medical Control.* New York: Praeger.
Ruzek, Sheryl Burt and Julie Becker. 1999. "The Women's Health Movement in the United States: From Grass-Roots Activism to Professional Agendas." *Journal of the American Medical Women's Association* 54:4–8.
Saks, Mike. 1983. "Removing the Blinkers? A Critique of Recent Contributions to the Sociology of Professions." *Sociological Review* 31:1–21.
Schecter, Kate. 2000. "The Politics of Health Care in Russia: The Feminization of Medicine and Other Obstacles to Professionalism." Pp. 83–99 in *Russia's Torn Safety Nets: Health and Social Welfare During the Transition,* edited by Mark G. Field and Judyth L. Twigg. New York: St. Martin's.
Schiøtz, Aina and Rannveig Nordhagen. 1992. "Om å sette sin kvinnelighet på spill: Kvinners adgang til det medisinske studium; Marie Spångberg og andre pionerer." *Tidsskrift for Den norske lægeforening* 112:3784–90.
Schondel, Annie and Kirsten Sølvsten Sørensen. 1984. "De første 50 år (1885–1934) og lidt af de næste." Pp. 13–53 in *I Nielsines fodspor: kvindelige læger gennem 100 år,* edited by Borum, K., B. Danneskiold-Samsøe, V. Jørgensen, A. Kjær, S. Kroon, A. Schondel, and K.S. Sørenson. Copenhagen: Munksgaard.
Schultz, Daniel S. and Michael P. Rafferty. 1990. "Soviet Health Care and Perestroika." *American Journal of Public Health* 80:193–97.
*Science.* 1995. Special issue on Women's health research. *Science* 269(August 11).
Seaman, Barbara. 1969. *The Doctors' Case Against the Pill.* New York: Peter H. Wyden.
Sheppard, Deborah L. 1989. "Organizations, Power and Sexuality: The Image and Self-Image of Women Managers." Pp. 139–57 in *The Sexuality of Organizations,* edited by Jeff Hearn, Deborah L. Sheppard, Peter Tancred-Sheriff, and Gibson Burrell. London: Sage.
Shumaker, Sally A. and Teresa Rust Smith. 1994. "The Politics of Women's Health." *Journal of Social Issues* 50:189–202.
Silverman, David. 1987. *Communication and Medical Practice: Social Relations in the Clinic.* London: Sage.
Simons, Kai and Carol Featherstone. 2000. "Science in Europe." *Science* 290:1099–1101.
Skard, Torild and Elina Haavio-Mannila. 1985. "Mobilization of Women at Elections." Pp. 37–50 in *Unfinished Democracy: Women in Nordic Politics.* Oxford: Pergamon.
Skocpol, Theda. 1992. *Protecting Soldiers and Mothers: The Political Origins of Social Policy in the United States.* Cambridge, M.A.: Harvard University Press.

Sobecks, Nancy W., Amy C. Justice, Susan Hinze, et. al. 1999. "When Doctors Marry Doctors: A Survey Exploring the Professional and Family Lives of Young Physicians." *Annals of Internal Medicine* 130:312–19.

Solomon, Susan Gross. 1990. "Social Hygiene and Soviet Public Health." Pp. 175–99 in *Health and Society in Revolutionary Russia*, edited by Susan Gross Solomon and John F. Hutchinson. Bloomington: Indiana University Press.

Sperling, Valerie. 2000. "The 'New' Sexism: Images of Russian Women during the Transition." Pp. 173–89 in *Russia's Torn Safety Nets: Health and Social Welfare during the Transition*, edited by Mark G. Field and Judyth L. Twigg. New York: St. Martin's Press.

Ståhle, Bertel. 1998. *Kvinder og maend i dansk universitetsforskning i 1990'erne.* Copenhagen: Undervisningsministeriet.

Starr, Paul. 1982. *The Social Transformation of American Medicine.* New York: Basic Books.

Stephens, John D. 1996. "The Scandinavian Welfare States: Achievements, Crisis and Prospects." Pp. 32–65 in: *Welfare States in Transition: National Adoptions in Global Economies*, edited by Gøsta Esping-Andersen. London: Sage.

Stevens, Rosemary. 1976. *American Medicine and the Public Interest.* New Haven, CT: Yale University Press.

Stevens, Rosemary. 1982. "A Poor Sort of Memory: Voluntary Hospitals before the Depression." *Milbank Memorial Quarterly* 60:551–84.

Stimson, Gerry V. 1985. "Recent Developments in Professional Control: The Impaired Physician Movement in the USA." *Sociology of Health and Illness* 7:141–66.

Stites, Richard. 1990. *The Women's Liberation Movement in Russia: Feminism, Nihilism and Bolshevism, 1860–1930.* Princeton, NJ: Princeton University Press.

Strauss, Anselm, Shizuko Fagerhaugh, Barbara Suczek, and Carolyn Wiener. 1985. *Social Organization of Medical Work.* Chicago: University of Chicago Press.

Suomen, Naislääkäriyhdistys. 1987. *Suomen Naislääkäriyhdistys r.y.—Finlands Kvinnliga Läkares Förening rf. 1947–1987.* Helsinki: Kaivopuiston kirjapaino oy.

Swedish Medical Association. 2000. *Swedish Physicians 2000* (leaflet). Stockholm.

Taylor, Verta. 1996. *Rock-a-by Baby: Feminism, Self-Help and Postpartum Depression.* New York: Routledge.

Tesch, Bonnie J., Helen M. Wood, Amy L. Helwig, and Ann Butler Nattinger. 1995. "Promotion of Women Physicians in Academic Medicine: Glass Ceiling or Sticky Floor?" *Journal of American Medical Association* 273:1022–25.

Thomas, Jan E. 1993. "Feminist Women's Health Centers: Internal Structures and External Forces." Paper presented at the annual meeting of the American Sociological Association in Miami Beach, Florida, August 13–17.

Thorne, Barrie. 1975. "Women in the Draft Resistance Movement: A Case Study of Sex Roles and Social Movements." *Sex Roles* 1:179–95.

Tocqueville, Alexis de. [1835] 1945. *Democracy in America* (Vol. 2). New York: Random House/Vintage.

Töyry, Saara, Kimmo Räsänen, Maria Hirvonen, et al. 2001. "Lääkärien työolot ja kuormittuneisuus: Taulukkoraportti." Finnish Medical Association: http://www.laakariliitto.fi/cgi/navi?.

Turner, Brian. 1997. "From Governmentality to Risk: Some Reflections on Foucault's Contribution to Medical Sociology." Pp. ix–xxi in *Foucault: Health and Medicine*, edited by Alan Petersen and Robin Bunton. London: Routledge.

Tuve, Jeanette. 1984. *The First Russian Women Physicians*. Newtonville, MA: Oriental Research Partners.
Twaddle, Andrew C. 1999. *Health Care Reform in Sweden, 1980–1994*. Westport, CT: Auburn House.
Twigg, Judyth L. 1999. "Obligatory Medical Insurance in Russia: The Participants' Perspective." *Social Science and Medicine* 49:371–82.
Twigg, Judyth L. 2000. "Unfulfilled Hopes: The Struggle to Reform Russian Health Care and Its Financing." Pp. 43–64 in *Russia's Torn Safety Nets: Health and Social Welfare during the Transition*, edited by Mark G. Field and Judyth L. Twigg. New York: St. Martin's.
U.S. Department of Health and Human Services. 1998. *Health, United States 1998, with Socioeconomic Status and Health Chartbook*. Washington, DC: USGPO.
Ulstad, Valerie K. 1993. "How Women Are Changing Medicine." *Journal of the American Medical Women's Association* 48:75–78.
van Elderen, T., S. Maes, C. Rouneau, and G. Seegers. 1998. "Perceived Gender Differences in Physician Consulting Behaviour during Internal Examination." *Family Practice* 15:147–52.
Vinder, K. 1975. *Kvinde, kend din krop*. Copenhagen: Tiderne skifter.
Vinder, K. [1975] 1983. *Kvinde, kend din krop* (2nd ed.). Copenhagen: Tiderne skifter.
Vinder, K. [1975] 1992 *Kvinde, kend din krop* (3rd ed.). Copenhagen: Tiderne skifter.
Wagner, David. 1997. *The New Temperance: The American Obsession with Sin and Vice*. Boulder, CO: Westview.
Walby, Sylvia. 1990. *Theorizing Patriarchy*. Oxford: Basil Blackwell.
Walsh, Mary Roth. 1977. *Doctors Wanted: No Women Need Apply: Sexual Barriers in the Medical Profession, 1835–1975*. New Haven, CT: Yale University Press.
Walsh, Mary Roth. 1990. "Women in Medicine since Flexner." *New York State Journal of Medicine* 90:302–8.
Weinstein, Eugene A. and Paul Deutschberger. 1963. "Some Dimensions of Alter Casting." *Sociometry* 26:454–66.
Weissman, Neil B. 1990. "Origins of Soviet Health Administration, Narkozdrav, 1918–1928." Pp. 97–120 in *Health and Society in Revolutionary Russia*, edited by Susan Gross Solomon and John F. Hutchinson. Bloomington: Indiana University Press.
Wennerås, Christine and Agnes Wold. 1997. "Nepotism and Sexism in Peer-Review." *Nature* 387:341–43.
West, Candace. 1993. "Reconceptualizing Gender in Physician-Patient Relationships." *Social Science and Medicine* 36:57–66.
West, Candace and Don H. Zimmerman. 1987. "Doing Gender." *Gender and Society* 1:125–51.
Westermarck, Helena. 1930. *Finlands första kvinnliga läkare: Rosina Heikel*. Helsingfors: Söderström.
Williams, A. Paul. 1999. "Changing the Palace Guard: Analysing the Impact of Women's Entry into Medicine." *Gender, Work and Organization* 6:106–21.
Williams, Christine L. 1992. "The Glass Escalator: Hidden Advantages for Men in the 'Female' Professions." *Social Problems* 39:253–67.
Wilsford, David. 1991. *Doctors and the State. The Politics of Health Care in France and the United States*. Durham, NC: Duke University Press.
Witz, Anne. 1992. *Professions and Patriarchy*. London: Routledge.
Witz, Anne. 2000. "Whose Body Matters? Feminist Sociology and the Corporeal Turn in Sociology and Feminism." *Body and Society* 6:1–24.

Wrong, Dennis H. 1961. "The Oversocialized Conception of Man in Modern Sociology." *American Sociological Review* 24:772–82.

Zimmer, Lynn. 1988. "Tokenism and Women in the Workplace." *Social Problems* 35:64–77.

Zimmerman, Mary. 1987. "The Women's Health Movement: A Critique of Medical Enterprise and the Position of Women." Pp. 442–72 in *Analyzing Gender: A Handbook of Social Science Research*, edited by Beth B. Hess and Myra Marx Ferree. Beverly Hills: Sage.

Zimmerman, Mary K. and Shirley A. Hill. 2000. "Reforming Gendered Health Care: An Assessment of Change." *International Journal of Health Services* 30: 771–95.

Zola, Irving K. 1972. "Medicine as an Institution of Social Control." *Sociological Review* 20:487–503.

# Index